FINE FOOD
FOR THE HEART

CHEREE MELLOW
& GLENDA ROBBIE

THE NATIONAL HEART FOUNDATION
OF NEW ZEALAND

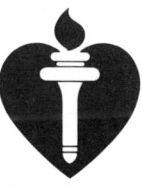

FOREWORD

ISBN 0-473-00527-1

FOREWORD

These days, many New Zealanders want healthier lifestyles.

They are exercising more and want to improve their eating habits, not just for a week or a month, but for a longer term.

The New Zealand Nutrition Guidelines advise a wide variety of foods, with special emphasis on plenty of foods high in fibre while taking care not to include too much fat, sugar and salt.

The National Heart Foundation's new recipe book explains how to put this into practice in an enjoyable way.

The recipes use fresh New Zealand ingredients to create interesting, healthy dishes which will have wide appeal to families as well as heart patients.

The book gives microwave as well as conventional cooking instructions, and lists kilojoules and calories per serving. It will help the cook who is looking for recipes and hints for all meals and courses, including packed lunches. The introduction includes advice on diet and prevention of heart disease.

Right through the book runs the message that variety and moderate amounts are the keys to healthy eating and a healthy heart!

Alison Holst

ACKNOWLEDGEMENTS

Authors: **Cheree Mellow**, B.H.Sc
Dietitian, National Heart
Foundation of New Zealand.

Glenda Robbie B.H.Sc. Dip Tchg.
Advanced Certificate Leith's School
of Food and Wine, London.
Consultant Home Economist.

Photography: Alan Gillard

Editor: Jill Pierce

**National Heart Foundation
Scientific Committee
Advisors:** Professor John Hunter, Chairman
Dr David Hay, Medical Director.

**Health Education
Committee Advisor:** Dr Peter Leslie, Chairman.

Design and Artwork: Aldous Creative Enterprises.

Typesetting: Jacobsons.

Printing: Through Aldous Creative Enterprises.

Published in 1987 by the National Heart Foundation
with the assistance of Caltex Oil (N.Z.) Ltd.

Distributed by Beckett Publishing.

CONTENTS

Standard level metric cup and
spoon measurements have been
used throughout this book.

Tbsp = tablespoon, tsp = teaspoon, g = gram,
kg = kilogram, kJ = kilojoule, cal = calorie,
1 metric cup = 250mls.

INTRODUCTION

Good eating habits based on variety and moderation combined with a healthy lifestyle may significantly reduce the risk of heart disease. The Heart Foundation promotes the benefits of a healthy lifestyle. A well-balanced diet with regular activity will maintain a healthy weight. Emphasis is given to increasing fibre content, and restricting the amounts of fat and cholesterol.

This recipe book is based on the **Nutrition Guidelines for New Zealanders** as well as meeting the Heart Foundation's recommendations. It aims to show that healthy eating can be enjoyable, economical and interesting for the whole family, no matter how young or how old. These guidelines are as follows:-

1. Eat a variety of foods.
2. Achieve and maintain weight within a healthy range.
3. Use only a little sugar.
4. Keep fat intake low.
5. Eat adequate food fibre.
6. Take care with salt.
7. Drink alcohol in moderation.

1. **Why a variety of foods?**
   There is no perfect food which supplies all the essential nutrients in the amounts you need to stay healthy. To achieve a well-balanced diet each day include:

   - **mainly** breads and cereals (especially wholegrain varieties) and fruits and vegetables
   - **moderate** amounts of
     – lean meat, poultry, fish, legumes (dried peas, beans and lentils) nuts and eggs
     – low fat dairy products (non-fat milk, low fat yoghurt and cottage cheese)
   - **small** amounts of
     – polyunsaturated margarine and vegetable oil
     – sugar and salt

2. **Keep a healthy weight.**
   Being overweight is associated with many health problems, such as high blood pressure and diabetes, which are also risk factors for coronary

heart disease. To lose weight it is important to increase physical activity by exercising regularly and decrease the energy (kilojoule) content of your diet. This means eating less fat and fatty food, less sugar and sugar containing foods and little or no alcohol. For weight conscious cooks the approximate kilojoule and calorie content of each recipe has been calculated.

3. **Use only a little sugar.**
   Although there is no direct relationship between eating sugar and developing heart disease, sugar is high in energy (kilojoules) and provides little else in the way of nutrients. A high intake of sugar can contribute to overweight. Foods high in sugar often contain very little fibre, making it easy to overeat these foods.

   To moderate your intake of sugar and foods with a high sugar content use less sugar (white, brown, raw, honey and syrups), and eat fewer cakes, sweet biscuits, confectionery and soft drinks.

   In our recipes we have not banished sugar altogether, but we have kept it to a moderate level. The sweetness in the desserts and baked foods is supplied by the natural sweetness of fruits and where necessary we have used tinned fruit with no added sugar.

4. **Keep fat intake low.**
   Fats are the most concentrated source of energy in the diet, and can also lead to being overweight.

   The average New Zealand diet is high in fat and cholesterol and the proportion of saturated fat (mainly animal fat) to polyunsaturated fat (mainly vegetable fat) is also very high. Such a diet tends to be associated with high blood fat levels, increasing the risk of heart disease.

   New Zealanders generally are advised to reduce their intake of total fat and cholesterol and replace some of the saturated fat by polyunsaturated fat. To reduce the fat content of the recipes in this book we have emphasised moderate portions of lean meat and chicken. Fish in all its forms features strongly. Full cream dairy products have been avoided, with many recipes using non-fat milk, low fat yoghurt and low fat cheeses such as cottage, ricotta, and small quantities of edam and parmesan cheese. The amount of fat used for cooking, or spreads, in salad dressings and sauces is limited. Where necessary we have used only small quantities of polyunsaturated margarines and vegetable oils instead of butter and other cooking fats. The recipes also encourage low fat cooking methods such as grilling, baking, steaming or microwaving in preference to frying.

5. **Eat adequate food fibre.**
Fibre is found in plant foods such as grains and cereal products, fruits and vegetables. Eating these foods can help control body weight – they are moderately low in energy (kilojoules) and the fibre provides bulk to help you feel full. Including extra fibre in the diet may also have a beneficial effect on blood fat levels. Choose a variety of different high fibre foods daily:

- Breads and cereal products (especially wholegrain varieties) like pasta and high fibre breakfast cereals.
- Wholegrains like brown rice, oats and barley
- Fruits and vegetables
- Legumes – dried peas, beans and lentils.
- Nuts and seeds (in moderation due to their high fat content).

6. **Take care with salt.**
Many New Zealanders eat more salt than they need, either as salt added to food during cooking and at the table, or in processed foods where salt is a preservative or a flavouring agent. Although not all high blood pressure is due to excess salt in the diet, there is good reason to believe that a reduced intake would be advisable, even just to appreciate the true flavour of food.

For seasoning in the book we have emphasised the use of fresh herbs and spices as replacements for salt. We have generally avoided processed foods containing large amounts of added salt, commercial sauces, stock cubes and soup powders. When shopping, look out for any new 'no added salt' products.

7. **Drink alcohol in moderation.**
Alcoholic drinks tend to be high in energy

(kilojoules) and low in other nutrients. Heavy drinkers also tend to neglect the rest of their diet. Small amounts of alcohol with meals as part of a varied diet may be harmless, but large amounts are clearly to be avoided.

There are a variety of recipes in this book, all of them imaginative and easy to prepare. The food is to be cooked quickly and simply to retain maximum flavour and nutritional value. The recipes are designed to be low in fat, sugar and salt and rich in fibre. Simplicity is our aim so that cooking can be fun without being arduous, and interesting without being too complicated. Remember to balance a good diet with a healthy active lifestyle. Variety and moderation go with healthy eating and a healthy heart.

THE HEALTHY FOOD PYRAMID

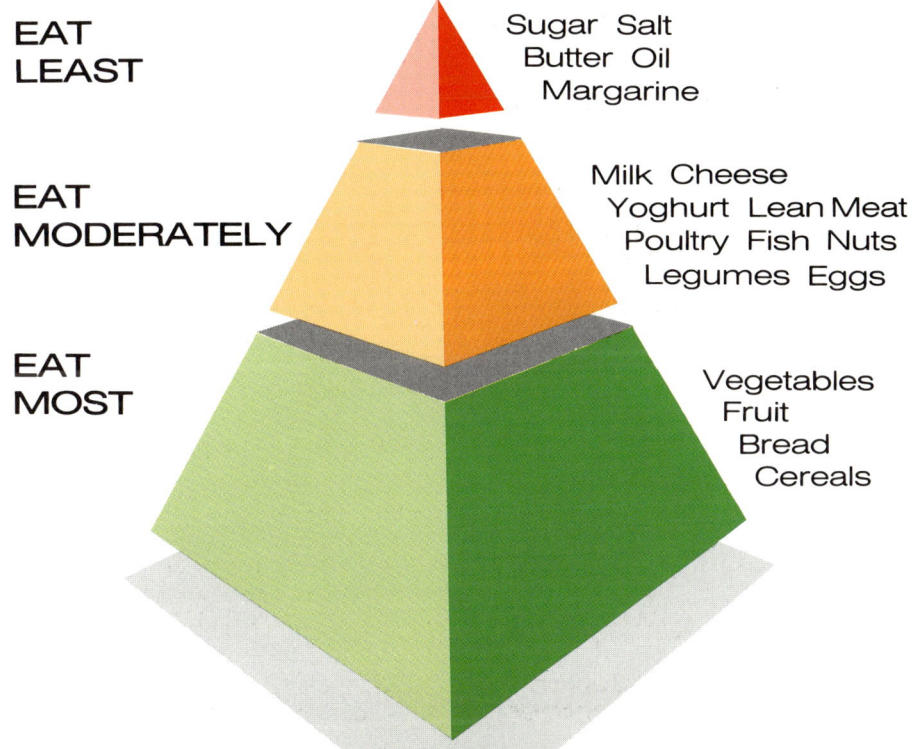

EAT LEAST — Sugar Salt Butter Oil Margarine

EAT MODERATELY — Milk Cheese Yoghurt Lean Meat Poultry Fish Nuts Legumes Eggs

EAT MOST — Vegetables Fruit Bread Cereals

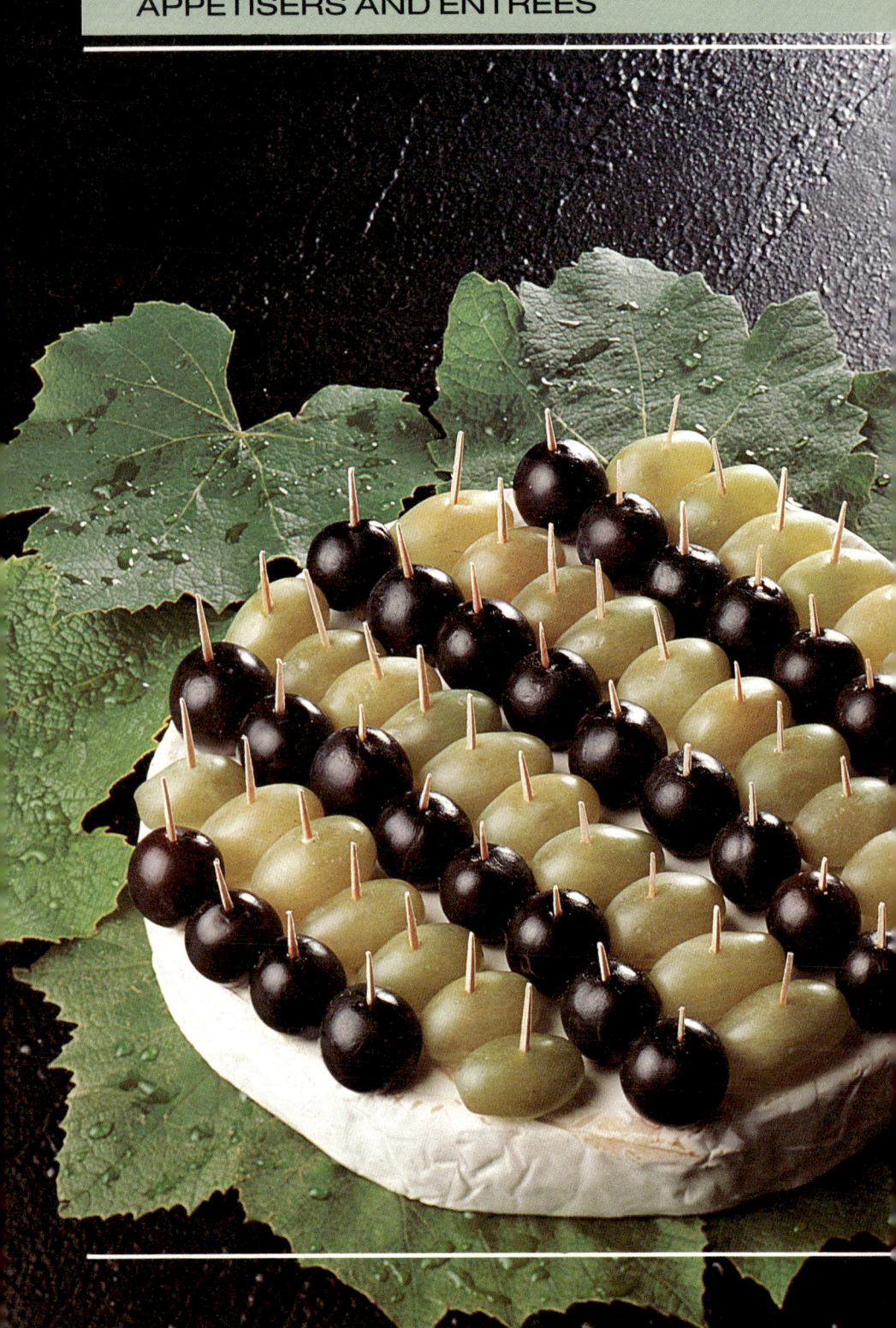

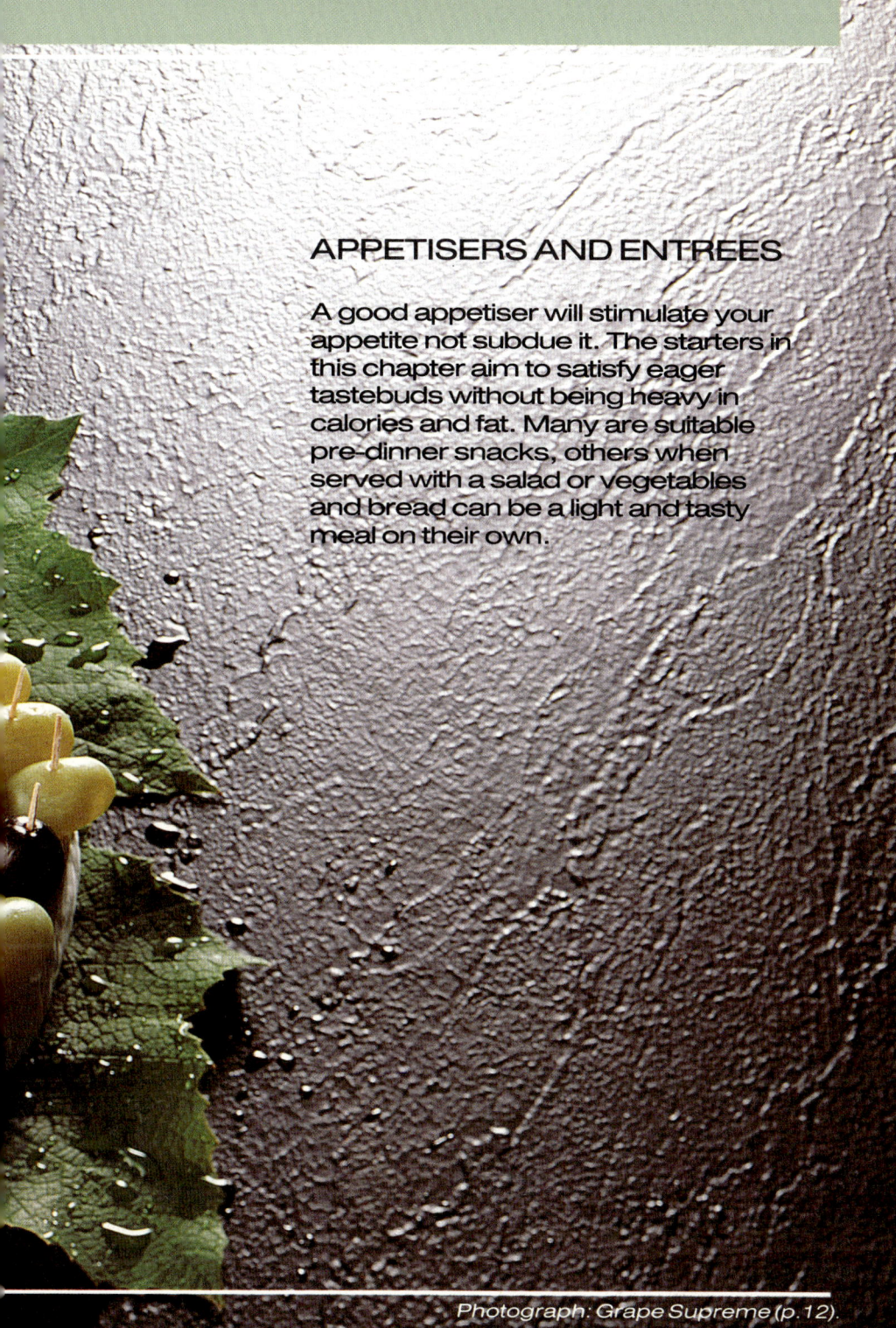

APPETISERS AND ENTREES

A good appetiser will stimulate your appetite not subdue it. The starters in this chapter aim to satisfy eager tastebuds without being heavy in calories and fat. Many are suitable pre-dinner snacks, others when served with a salad or vegetables and bread can be a light and tasty meal on their own.

Photograph: Grape Supreme (p.12).

CHEESEY BITES

The savoury flavour of cheese is especially attractive at the start of a meal. This recipe teams a moderately low fat cheese with dried fruit, to make a popular finger food.

70g edam cheese
20 pitted prunes
   or dates

Cut the cheese into 20 small cubes. Split each prune or date and place a cube of cheese in the split. Bake at 180°C for 5-8 minutes or until the cheese begins to melt. Serve hot.
[90 kJ (21 Cal) per Cheesy Bite]

Microwave
Cover with plastic film and cook on 100% power for 1-1½ minutes or until the cheese begins to melt. Serve hot.

GRAPE SUPREME

We have illustrated a brie which would be suitable for serving a group of about 12-15 people. The standard sized brie or camembert would serve approximately 5-6 for cocktails.

1 brie or camembert
   cheese
green grapes
black grapes

Select a brie or camembert which is soft. Arrange rows of grapes alternating between green and black. Secure in place with toothpicks. Cut the cheese into cubes so as each cube has a grape on top. Serve as a complete wheel of cheese.
[202 kJ (48 Cal) per cube]

Photograph page 10.

FILO TRIANGLES

Filo pastry is an excitingly different type of pastry — flakey and light (and low in fat) it is ideal for the start of a meal.

8 sheets filo pastry
3 Tbsp polyunsaturated
  oil
1 tsp sesame seeds

Lay one sheet of pastry on a clean, flat surface and brush sparingly with oil. Place the next sheet on top of this. Cut into quarter widths. Place one tablespoon of the chosen filling at one end and fold end over to form a triangle. Continue folding up the length to make a layered, triangular parcel. Sprinkle with sesame seeds. Repeat until all pastry and filling is used up. Bake at 200°C for 20 minutes or until golden brown. Serve hot.
Makes 16 triangles. [323 kJ (77 Cal) per triangle]

Suggested fillings

Courgette and Mint

3 cups grated courgette
2 Tbsp finely chopped
  fresh mint
2 Tbsp finely chopped
  walnuts
3 Tbsp natural low fat
  cottage cheese

Squeeze the courgettes to remove as much of the juices as possible. Mix the courgettes, mint, walnuts and cottage cheese together.

Crab and Dill

6 crabsticks
1 Tbsp finely chopped
  fresh dill
⅓ cup natural low fat
  yoghurt
2 Tbsp lemon juice
freshly ground black
  pepper

Chop the crabsticks finely. Mix the crab, dill, yoghurt, lemon juice and pepper together.

PUMPERNICKEL PLATTER

Pumpernickel is a dark rye bread, low in fat and high in fibre. Available already sliced, it is moist yet firm enough to be an ideal base for toppings.

pumpernickel bread

Topping 1:
natural low fat cottage
   cheese
peeled and sliced
   kiwifruit
fresh dill
finely diced red, green
   and yellow pepper

Topping 2:
ricotta cheese
raspberry halves
grated lemon rind
sliced spring onion

Topping 3:
mashed hard
   boiled egg
peeled and sliced
   green grapes
diced yellow pepper
fresh thyme

Topping 4:
celery leaves
celery slices
sliced edam cheese
finely sliced red pepper
alfalfa sprouts

Cut the pumpernickel into bite-sized squares.
Top with suggested toppings as illustrated or
experiment with other combinations eg.
— ricotta cheese, melon and mint
— natural low fat cottage cheese, pickled onion, red
pepper and watercress
—quark, strawberry and gherkin
— egg, parsley and radish
  [92 kJ (22 Cal) per slice pumpernickel].

Photograph opposite page

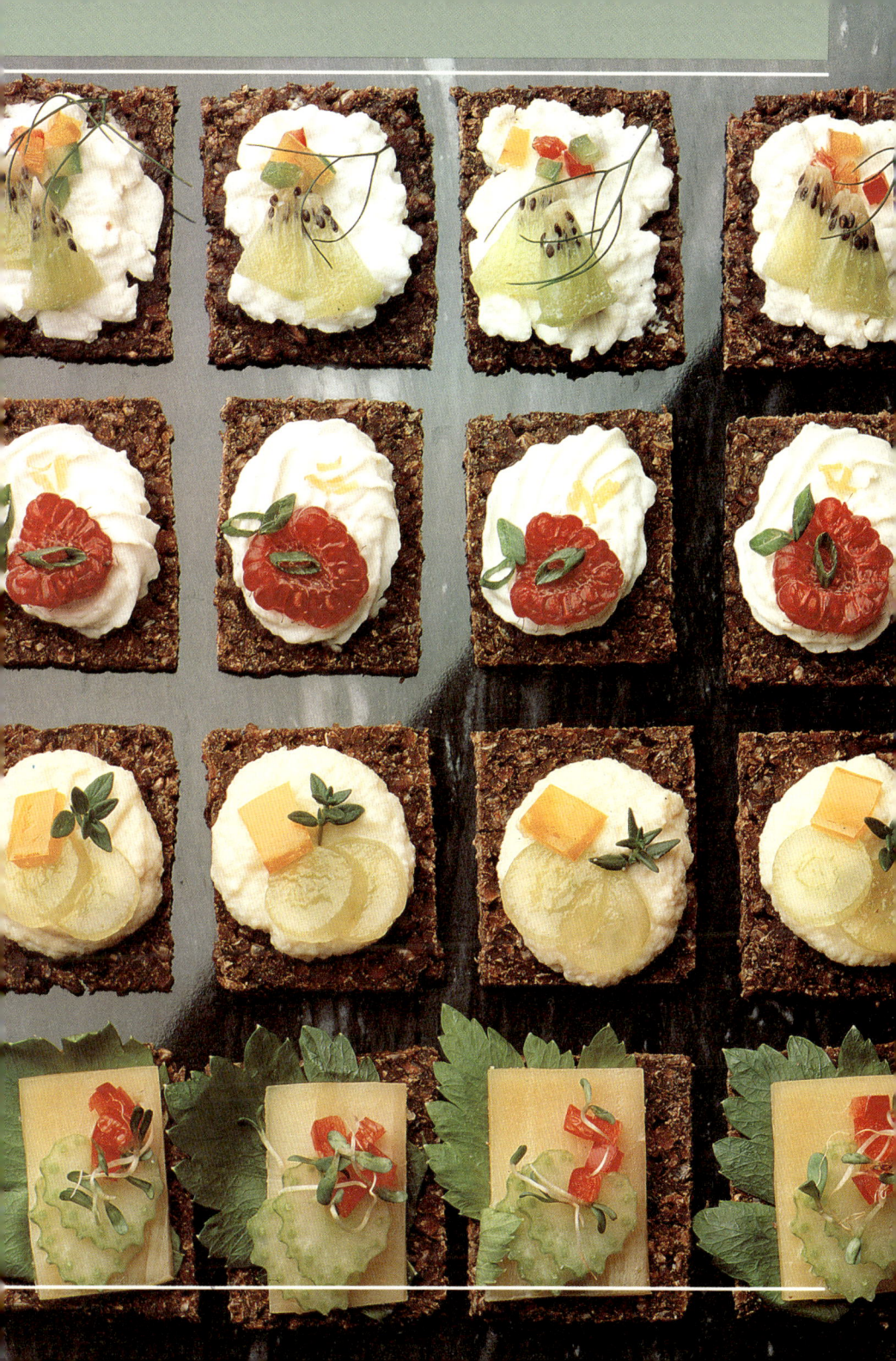

AVOCADO WITH ORANGE DRESSING

The smooth texture and rich flavour of the avocado contrasts well with the tangy orange dressing. Avocados are high in vegetable oils, so remember they are also high in calories. Keep this recipe for special occasions.

3 avocados
orange slices for
   garnish

Cut the avocado in half lengthwise and remove the stone and skin. Place the cut side down on a board. Cut slices 1cm wide, starting 2cm down from the top and cutting to the base. Press gently to fan the slices out. Transfer to a serving plate. Pour over the dressing. Garnish with orange slices.
Serves 6. [714 kJ (170 Cal) per serving)

Orange Dressing

1 orange
1 clove garlic, peeled
2 Tbsp white wine
   vinegar

2 Tbsp roughly
   chopped fresh
   oregano or chives
freshly ground black
   pepper

Using a sharp knife, remove the rind from the orange taking as little pith as possible. Squeeze to give ½ cup juice. With the motor running drop the garlic and orange rind down the tube of a food processor fitted with a metal blade. Process until finely chopped. Add the orange juice, vinegar, herbs and pepper. Process until smooth. Chill.

BACON AND GARLIC DIP WITH PITA CHIPS

This dip recipe keeps the fat content down by using low fat dairy products. Serve it with wholemeal pita chips — high fibre, low salt alternatives to cocktail biscuits.

2 rashers lean bacon
1 clove garlic, peeled
    and finely chopped
3 spring onions, thinly
    sliced

2-3 Tbsp non-fat milk
1 cup natural low fat
    cottage cheese
freshly ground black
    pepper

Remove rind and all visible fat from the bacon. Grill until crisp and drain on absorbent paper. Chop finely. Mix the bacon, garlic, spring onions, milk and cottage cheese together. Season to taste with pepper. Serve with pita chips.
Makes approximately 1 cup. [2006 kJ (478 Cal) per recipe]

Microwave
Place trimmed bacon between paper towels. Cook on 100% power for 2-4 minutes. Chop finely.

Pita Chips

3 large pita breads

Cut each pita bread into 2cm wide strips. Cut these into 6cm long lengths. Split into single layers. Bake at 180°C for 10 minutes or until crisp and golden brown. Cool before serving. Store in an airtight container. [1175 kJ (280 Cal) per pita bread]

FISH TIMBALES ON TOMATO SAUCE

This recipe makes a striking and attractive first course. Served with a vegetable or salad it could also be a satisfying main meal.

300 g white fish fillets
  e.g. cod
¼ cup natural low fat
  yoghurt

freshly ground black
  pepper
2 egg whites
fresh basil for garnish

Tomato Sauce

300 g tin whole peeled
  tomatoes, undrained
  or 500g fresh
  tomatoes
1 onion, roughly
  chopped
1 carrot, roughly
  chopped

1 tsp dried basil or 1
  Tbsp chopped fresh
  basil
2 Tbsp tomato paste
freshly ground black
  pepper

Fish Timbales

Place the fish, yoghurt, and pepper in a food processor fitted with a metal blade. Process until evenly mixed. Whip the egg whites and fold into the fish mixture. Turn into 4 lightly greased ramekin dishes or cups. Cover with foil and place in a pan of water. Bake at 190°C for 12-15 minutes or until set. Invert onto a serving plate. Serve with the tomato sauce, garnished with fresh basil.

Tomato Sauce

If using fresh tomatoes, blanch and remove skins. Place the tomatoes, onion, carrot, basil, tomato paste and pepper in a saucepan. Simmer 15-20 minutes or until the onion softens. Puree until smooth.
Serves 4 [570 kJ (136 Cal) per serve].

Microwave

Place the tomatoes, onion, carrot, basil, tomato paste and pepper in a microwave proof dish and cook on 100% power for 10 minutes. Puree. Cover the fish timables with plastic film and cook on 70% power for 7-8 minutes.

MUSHROOM CAPS

Appetising and light, the spiced pineapple stuffing does not overpower the delicate flavour of the mushrooms.

30 medium sized mushrooms
1 cup drained, unsweetened crushed pineapple
½ tsp garam masala

1 egg
¼ cup finely chopped red or green pepper
½ cup fresh wholemeal breadcrumbs
freshly ground black pepper

Wash the mushrooms, peel if necessary. Remove the stalks and discard. Mix the pineapple, garam masala, egg, red or green pepper, breadcrumbs and ground pepper together. Place a spoonful of the mixture in each mushroom cap. Bake at 180°C for 10-15 minutes or until golden brown and the mushrooms are soft. Serve hot.
[85 kJ (20 Cal) per mushroom].

Note: If garam masala is not available, substitute with ground coriander.

Microwave

Cover and cook on 100% power for 5-6 minutes. Stand 4 minutes.

GINGER MELON BALLS

The fresh flavour of chilled melon combines well with the subtle taste of ginger — a light and appetising start to a meal.

3 pieces crystallised
 ginger
2 medium sized
 melons (eg. rock,
 prince)

¼ cup green ginger
 wine
fresh mint for garnish

Soak the crystallised ginger in boiling water for 5 minutes to remove the sugar. Drain and chop finely. Cut the melons in half and discard the seeds. Using a melon baller, scoop the melon into balls and place in a bowl. Reserve the juice and mix with the green ginger wine and ginger. Pour over the melon balls. Marinate in the refrigerator for at least 2 hours before serving. Serve chilled, garnished with mint.
Serves 4 [395 kJ (94 Cal) per serve].

Variation: A small watermelon may be used in place of the rock or prince melon.

Photograph opposite page

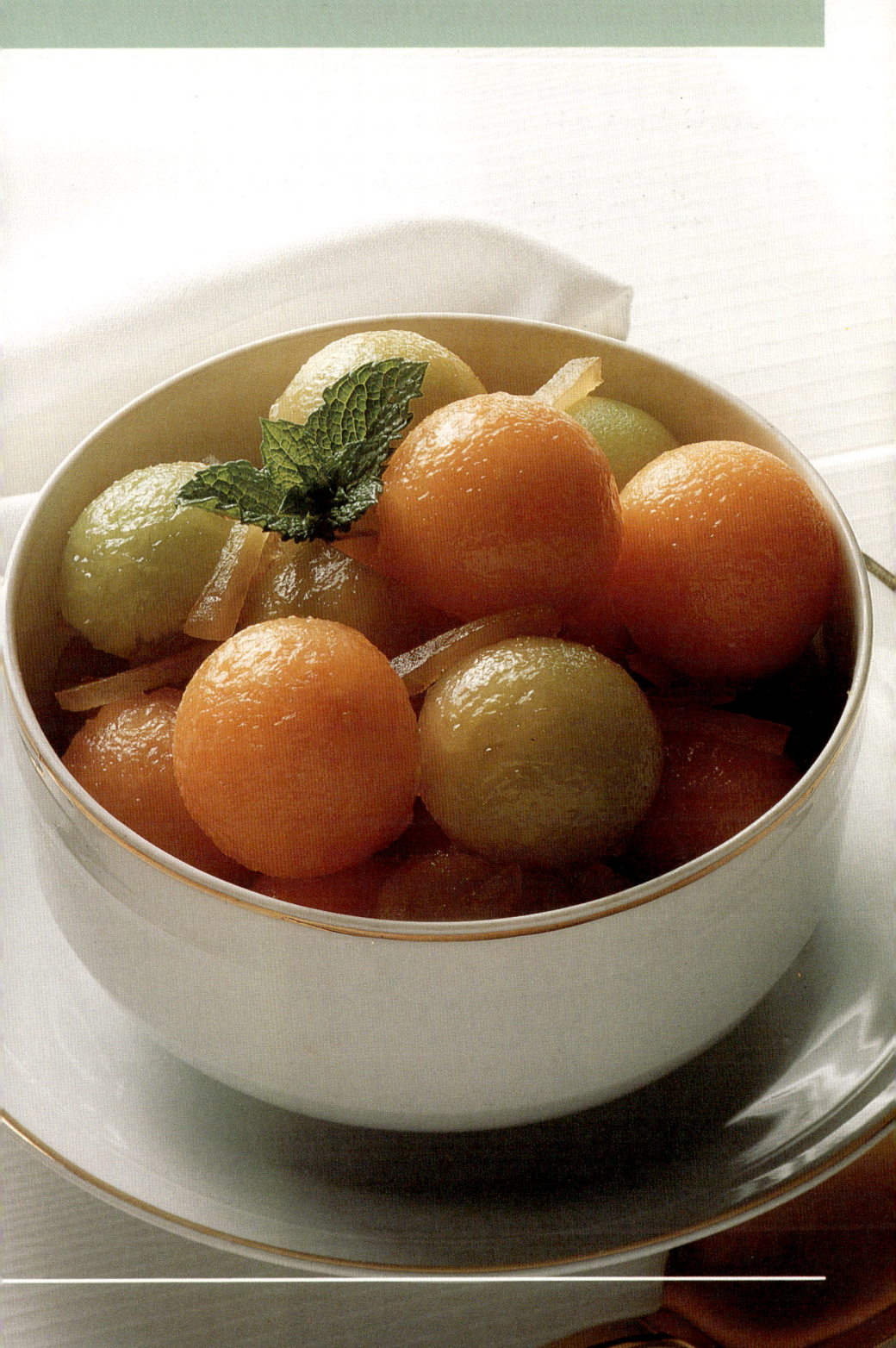

CELERY DIP

Dips are fun to serve, easy to make and enjoyed even by people who normally avoid salads or raw vegetables.

1 cup natural low fat
   cottage cheese
2 Tbsp grated
   parmesan cheese
½ cup roughly
   chopped celery

1 Tbsp lemon juice
¼-½ tsp tabasco
   sauce
1 Tbsp non-fat milk
   freshly ground black
   pepper

Place all ingredients in a food processor fitted with a metal blade and blend until smooth. Add extra milk if thinner consistency is preferred. Refrigerate before serving. Serve with crackers or crudites such as celery and carrot sticks, radish wedges, broccoli and cauliflower florets.
Makes approximately 1½ cups [1423 kJ (339 Cal) per recipe].

GRILLED GRAPEFRUIT

Grapefruit need not be served for breakfast only — this excellent source of vitamin C provides a refreshing entree.

2 grapefruit
2 Tbsp orange liqueur

1 Tbsp brown sugar
fresh mint for garnish

Cut each grapefruit in half. Using a grapefruit knife loosen the segments from the pith. Remove as much pith as possible. Pour the orange liqueur on each grapefruit half and sprinkle with brown sugar. Grill 5-10 minutes or until the grapefruit begins to brown. Serve hot, garnished with mint.
Serves 4 [331 kJ (79 Cal) per serve].

CHEESE LOG

This recipe's main contribution, apart from its velvety texture, is the hint of ginger which combines so well with the cheese. Suitable also as a filling for celery sticks.

1 cup natural low fat
   cottage cheese
50 g edam cheese

3-4 pieces crystallised
   ginger
3 Tbsp poppy seeds

Place the cottage cheese, edam cheese and ginger in a food processor fitted with a metal blade. Process until the cheese is finely chopped. Chill well. Shape into a 15cm long log. Roll in poppy seeds. Serve chilled with crackers or crudites. Makes 1 log. [2047 kJ (487 Cal) per recipe]

Photograph page 171.

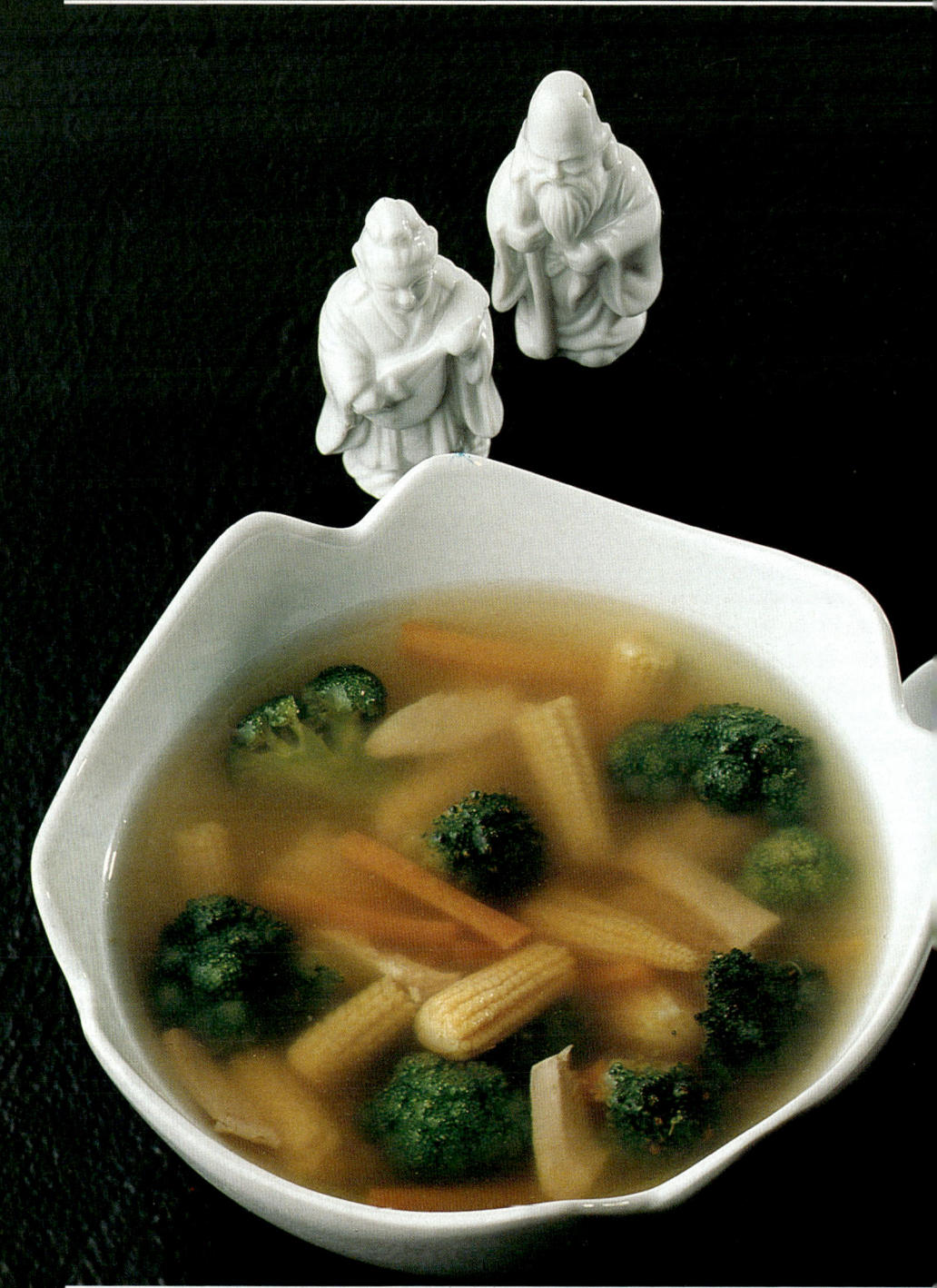

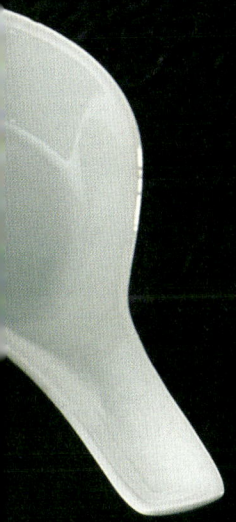

SOUPS

Soups are nutritious and delicious introductions to meals or meals in themselves. This chapter offers a wide selection of easy to prepare soups, thick and satisfying for winter, light and clear for summer and refreshing chilled soups for the end of a hot day. We have watched the amount of salt added, encouraging the use of homemade stocks and a variety of herbs and spices to give added flavour.

Photograph: Chinese Style Soup (p.27).

CHICKEN STOCK

Commercial stock cubes and powders have a high salt content. Homemade stocks are economical, tasty and can be kept in the freezer for later use.

2 chicken pieces
2 stalks celery,
    including leaves
2 carrots

2 unpeeled onions
3 bay leaves
6 cups water

Remove the skin and visible fat from the chicken. Roughly chop the celery, carrots and onions. Place in a large saucepan with the chicken, bay leaves and water. Cover and simmer gently for 1 hour. Cool and strain the stock. Remove chicken meat from the bones. This meat can be used elsewhere, such as in Chinese Style Soup. Chill the stock overnight and skim off all fat. Add sufficient water to make the volume of stock up to 6 cups. If not required immediately, freeze the undiluted stock and dilute once thawed.
Makes 6 cups.

Microwave
Cover and cook on 100% power for 25-30 minutes.

VEGETABLE STOCK

A good tasty stock is so important when making a successful soup. For a stock full of flavour and low in salt make your own from fresh vegetables and herbs rather than using commercial varieties.

2 unpeeled onions
2 carrots
6 stalks celery,
    including leaves
1 small turnip

5-6 sprigs fresh herbs
    eg. parsley, chives,
    thyme or 1 tsp dried
    mixed herbs
6-8 peppercorns
6 cups water

Roughly chop the onions, carrots, celery and turnip. Place in a large saucepan with herbs, peppercorns and water. Cover and simmer gently for 1 hour. Cool and strain the stock. Discard the vegetables. Add sufficient water to make the volume of stock up to 6 cups. If not required immediately, freeze the undiluted stock and dilute once thawed.
Makes 6 cups.

Microwave
Cover and cook on 100% power for 25-30 minutes.

CHINESE STYLE SOUP

A flavoursome stock is important. This soup is light and refreshing and makes a good balance with a satisfying main course.

6 cups chicken stock
   and reserved chicken
   meat (p 26)
3 carrots, finely sliced

2 cups broccoli florets
420 g tin baby corn
freshly ground black
   pepper

Place the stock, carrots, broccoli and drained baby corn in a saucepan. Cover and simmer for 20 minutes. Add the chicken meat. Simmer 5-10 minutes. Season generously with pepper.
Serves 6 [354 kJ (85 Cal) per serve].

Microwave
Place the stock, carrots, broccoli and drained baby corn in a microwave proof bowl. Cover and cook on 100% power for 15 minutes. Add the chicken and cook on 100% power for 3-4 minutes.

Photograph page 24

CHICKEN AND KUMARA SOUP

Kumara being naturally sweet, adds body and flavour to this soup. The non-fat milk helps to keep the fat content down.

1 quantity chicken
    stock and reserved
    chicken meat (p 26)
1 cup chopped celery
2 medium kumara,
    peeled and roughly
    chopped

1 cup non-fat milk
freshly ground black
    pepper

Do not dilute the chicken stock as instructed on p , boil to reduce to 3 cups. Place the stock, celery and kumara in a large saucepan. Cover and simmer for 30-35 minutes or until the vegetables are tender. Stir in the milk and chicken. Season to taste with pepper and re-heat.
Serves 4 [600 kJ (143 Cal) per serve].

Microwave
Cover and cook on 100% power for 18-20 minutes or until the vegetables are tender. Add the chicken, milk and pepper. Cook on 100% power for 2-3 minutes.

PARSNIP AND APPLE SOUP

This soup offers an unusual combination of flavours. Delicious and satisfying yet low in calories.

2 medium parsnips
2 apples
1 onion
6 cups chicken stock
    (p 26)

2 tsp curry powder
freshly ground black
    pepper
1/2 cup natural low fat
    yoghurt

Peel and finely chop the parsnips, apples and onion. Place in a saucepan with the stock, curry powder and pepper. Cover and simmer for 35-40 minutes.or until the vegetables are tender. Remove from the heat and stir in the yoghurt. Puree if wished.
Serves 6 [225 kJ (54 Cal) per serve].

Microwave
Cover and cook on 100% power for 20-25 minutes or until the parsnip is tender.

GINGERED CARROT SOUP

The ginger adds a wonderful freshness to this soup. Carrots provide vitamin A and their own natural sweetness. Simple and quick to prepare.

6 medium carrots,
  roughly chopped
2 medium potatoes,
  roughly chopped
4 cups chicken stock
  (p 26)

¼ tsp ground ginger
½ cup natural low fat
  yoghurt
freshly ground black
  pepper

Place the carrots, potatoes, stock and ginger in a saucepan. Cover and simmer for 20-25 minutes or until the vegetables are tender. Do not drain, puree until smooth. Stir in the yoghurt. Season to taste with pepper.
Serves 6 [225 kJ (54 Cal) per serve].

Microwave
Cover and cook on 100% power for 15-20 minutes or until the vegetables are tender.

Photograph page 31.

CURRIED CORN AND RICE SOUP

Full of fibre from the corn and rice, this is a thick, satisfying soup. When served with wholegrain bread and fresh fruit it provides a well-balanced meal without much effort.

2 rashers lean bacon
1 Tbsp polyunsaturated
   oil
1 onion, finely chopped
1½ tsp curry powder
1 Tbsp flour
1 cup non-fat milk
3 cups chicken stock
   (p 26)

½ cup rice
1 carrot, finely chopped
450 g tin whole kernel
   corn
2 Tbsp finely chopped
   fresh parsley
freshly ground black
   pepper

Remove the rind and visible fat from the bacon. Chop finely. Heat the oil in a heavy based saucepan and saute the bacon, onion and curry powder for 2-3 minutes. Add the flour and stir well. Gradually add the milk and stir continuously until the sauce thickens. Remove from the heat. Bring the chicken stock to the boil and add the rice. Cover and simmer for 15-20 minutes or until the rice is tender, add the carrot and drained corn. Continue simmering 10 minutes or until the carrots soften. Add the curry sauce, stir in the parsley and season with pepper. Reheat but do not boil.
Serves 6 [648 kJ (154 Cal) per serve].

Microwave

Cook the oil, bacon, onion and curry powder on 100% power for 3 minutes. Add the flour and stir well. Blend in the milk. Cook on 100% power for 3-4 minutes. Stir once during cooking. Cook the stock on 100% power for 4-5 minutes. Stir in the rice and cook on 100% power for 8-10 minutes. Stir in the carrot and drained corn. Cook on 100% power for 3-4 minutes or until the rice is tender. Add the curry sauce and parsley, season with pepper. Cook on 100% power for 2 minutes.

Photograph opposite page

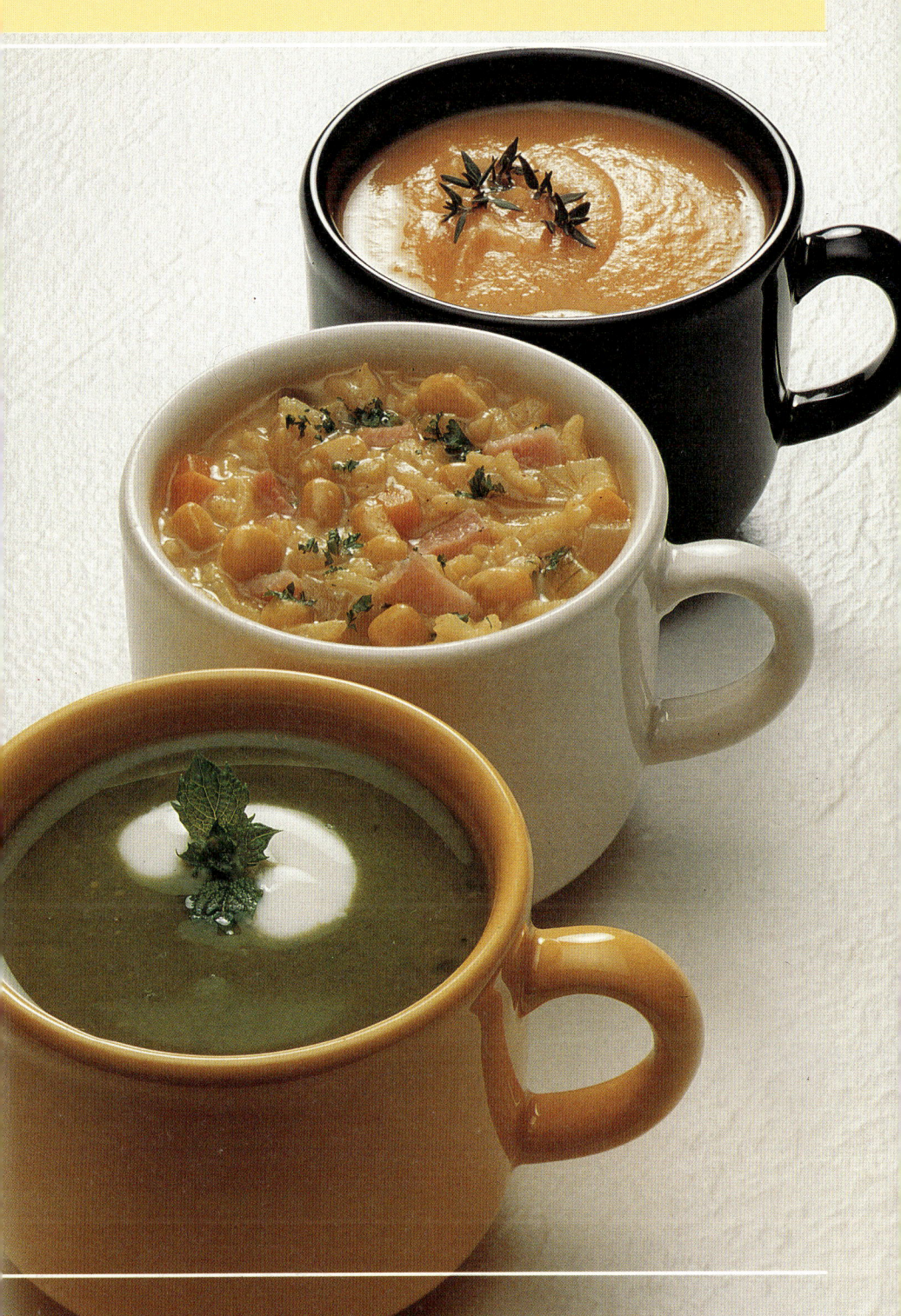

CHUNKY BEAN SOUP

This bean soup is delicious and satisfying as well as nutritious. Economical and easy to prepare, the beans provide protein, fibre, vitamins and minerals, yet are low in fat. A thick substantial soup — a meal in itself.

½ cup dried beans
1 onion, finely chopped
4 cups vegetable stock
  (p 26)
1 carrot, finely chopped

2 stalks celery, finely
  chopped
2 Tbsp tomato paste
3 Tbsp finely chopped
  fresh parsley
freshly ground black
  pepper

Soak the beans in water overnight, drain. In a large saucepan place the beans, onion and stock. Cover and simmer for 1 hour. Skim off any floating bean skins. Add the carrot, celery and tomato paste. Cook for a further 20-30 minutes or until the beans are tender. Stir in the parsley and season with pepper.
Serves 6 [302 kJ (72 Cal) per serve].

Microwave

Place the soaked and drained beans, onion and stock in a microwave proof bowl. Cover and cook on 100% power for 20 minutes. Add the carrot, celery and tomato paste. Cook on 100% power for 8-10 minutes. Stir in the parsley and season with pepper.

MINTED PEA SOUP

Pureed vegetables give soup a rich creamy texture without adding fat and calories. The subtle mint flavour adds freshness to this economical and tasty soup.

1 onion, finely chopped
3 cups chicken stock
  (p 26)
3 cups peas, fresh
  or frozen
1 Tbsp roughly
  chopped fresh
  majoram

¼ cup roughly
  chopped fresh mint
freshly ground black
  pepper
Garnish:
  natural low fat
  yoghurt
  fresh mint

Place the onion, stock, peas, majoram and mint in a saucepan. Cover and simmer for 20-25 minutes or until the onion is tender. Do not drain, puree until smooth. Season generously with pepper. Garnish with yoghurt and mint.
Serves 6 [196 kJ (47 Cal) per serve].

Microwave
Cover and cook on 100% power for 15-20 minutes or until the onion is tender.

Photograph page 31.

CHILLED CUCUMBER SOUP

Chilled soups can be a refreshing end to a hot day. To keep the fat content low in this soup use natural low fat yoghurt.

30cm cucumber
3 cups natural low fat
   yoghurt
3 sprigs fresh mint

Garnish:
fresh mint leaves
unpeeled cucumber
   slices

Peel the cucumber, remove seeds and roughly chop. Place the cucumber, yoghurt and mint in a food processor fitted with a metal blade. Blend until smooth. Serve chilled. Garnish with mint and cucumber slices.
Serves 6 [304 kJ (72 Cal) per serve].

CHILLED FRUIT SOUP

The pureed fruit in this recipe gives the soup a smooth creamy texture, yet is low in fat and surprisingly filling.

1 kg peeled and
   chopped stone fruit
   eg plums, peaches,
   apricots, nectarines
½ cup natural low fat
   yoghurt

Garnish:
natural low fat
   yoghurt
fruit slices

Place the chopped fruit and yoghurt in a food processor fitted with a metal blade. Blend until smooth. Add water if a thinner consistency is preferred. Chill well. Serve garnished with a swirl of yoghurt and a slice of the chosen fruit.
Serves 4 [496 kJ (118 Cal) per serve].

Variation: This soup is also delicious with berryfruit such as raspberries, boysenberries and strawberries.

Photograph opposite page.

Photograph: Chilled Fruit Soup (above).

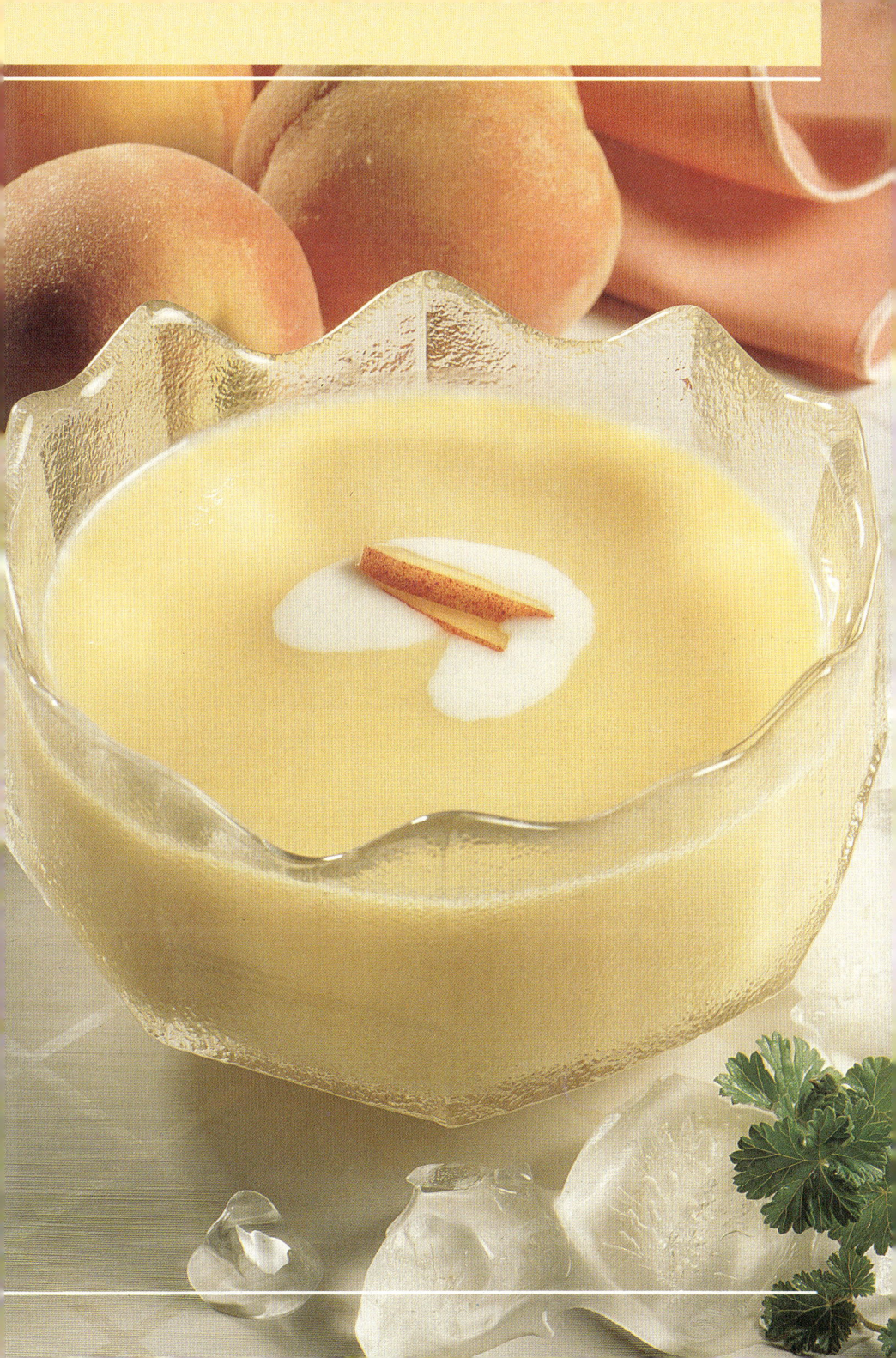

CUCUMBER AND TOMATO TWIN SOUP

Sure to impress your dinner guests, this attractive soup is not difficult. The secret is to ensure both soups are of a similar consistency.

½ quantity Chilled Cucumber Soup (p 34)
½ quantity Fresh Tomato and Basil Soup (p 37)

Prepare the soups as instructed. Each soup needs to be of a similar consistency, so adjust the Cucumber Soup with non-fat milk and the Tomato Soup with extra vegetable stock to achieve thick but pourable soups. Pour each soup into a jug and pour simultaneously into each soup bowl. Take care to pour at the same time and at the same rate. Serve chilled.
Serves 6 [205 kJ (49 Cal) per serve].

BLUE CHEESE AND PEAR SOUP

Although the blue cheeses are high in salt and fat, only a very small amount is needed to give a rich and creamy soup.

2 cups roughly
    chopped leeks
2 cups roughly
    chopped unpeeled
    pears
3 cups vegetable stock
    (p 26)
50g blue vein cheese
freshly ground black
    pepper

Place the leeks, pears and stock in a large saucepan. Cover and simmer for 20-25 minutes or until the leeks are tender. Add the blue cheese and pepper. Puree until smooth. Reheat but do not boil.
Serves 4 [620 kJ (148 Cal) per serve].

Microwave
Cover and cook on 100% power for 15-20 minutes or until the leeks are tender.

FRESH TOMATO AND BASIL SOUP

Served hot or cold, this tomato soup has a rich smooth character yet is low in calories and fat free — a suitable introduction to a meal in any season.

1 kg tomatoes or 2x400g tins whole peeled tomatoes, undrained
1 onion, roughly chopped
3 stalks celery, roughly chopped
4 bay leaves
2 cups vegetable stock (p 26)
2 Tbsp chopped fresh basil or 1 tsp dried basil
freshly ground black pepper

If using fresh tomatoes, blanch to remove skins. Roughly chop. Place tomatoes, onion, celery, bay leaves, stock, basil and pepper in a saucepan. Simmer gently for 25-30 minutes or until the onion is tender. Remove the bay leaves and puree. Add more stock if necessary to achieve preferred consistency. Serve hot or chilled.
Serves 6 [105 kJ (25 Cal) per serve].

Microwave
Cook on 100% power for 18-20 minutes.

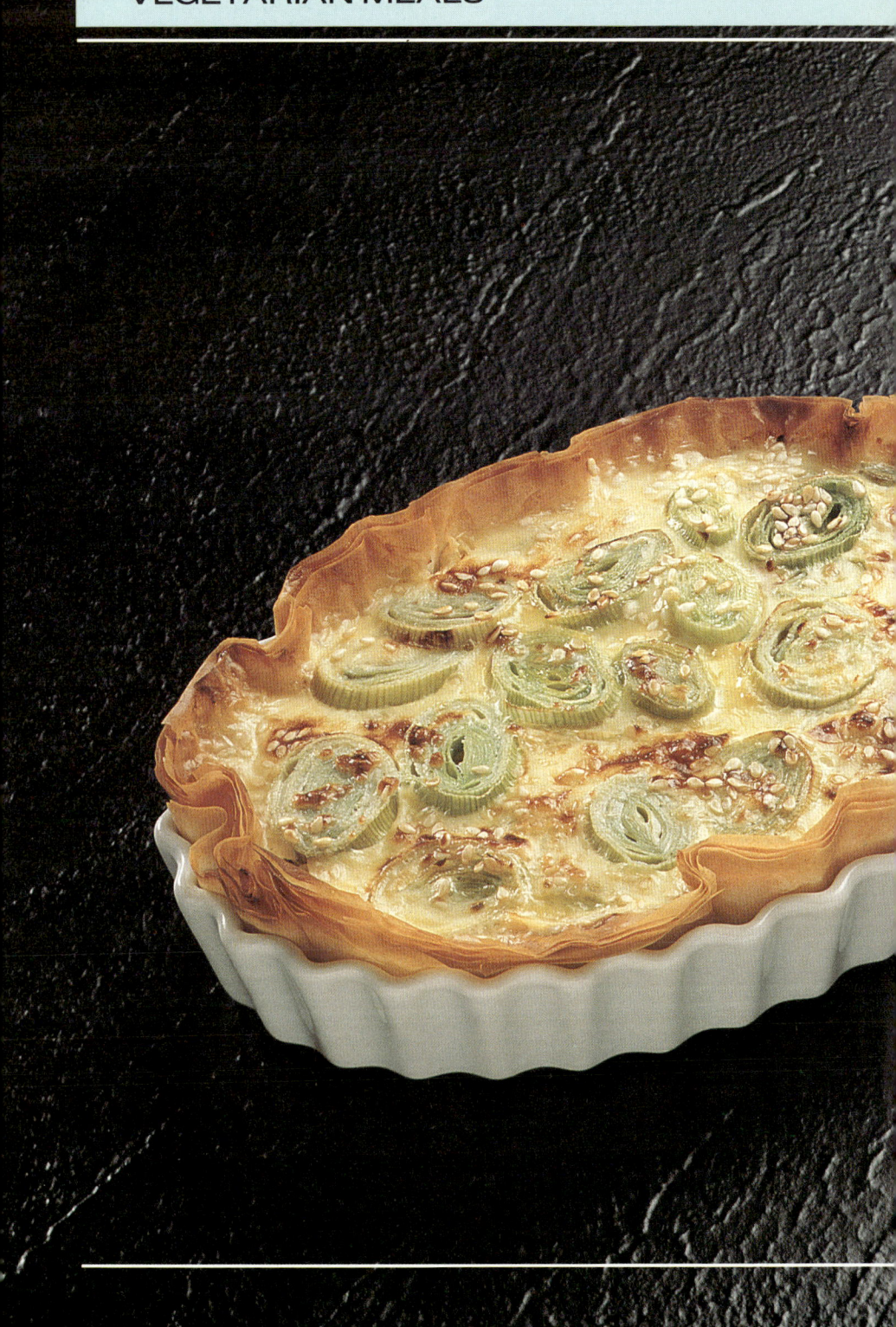

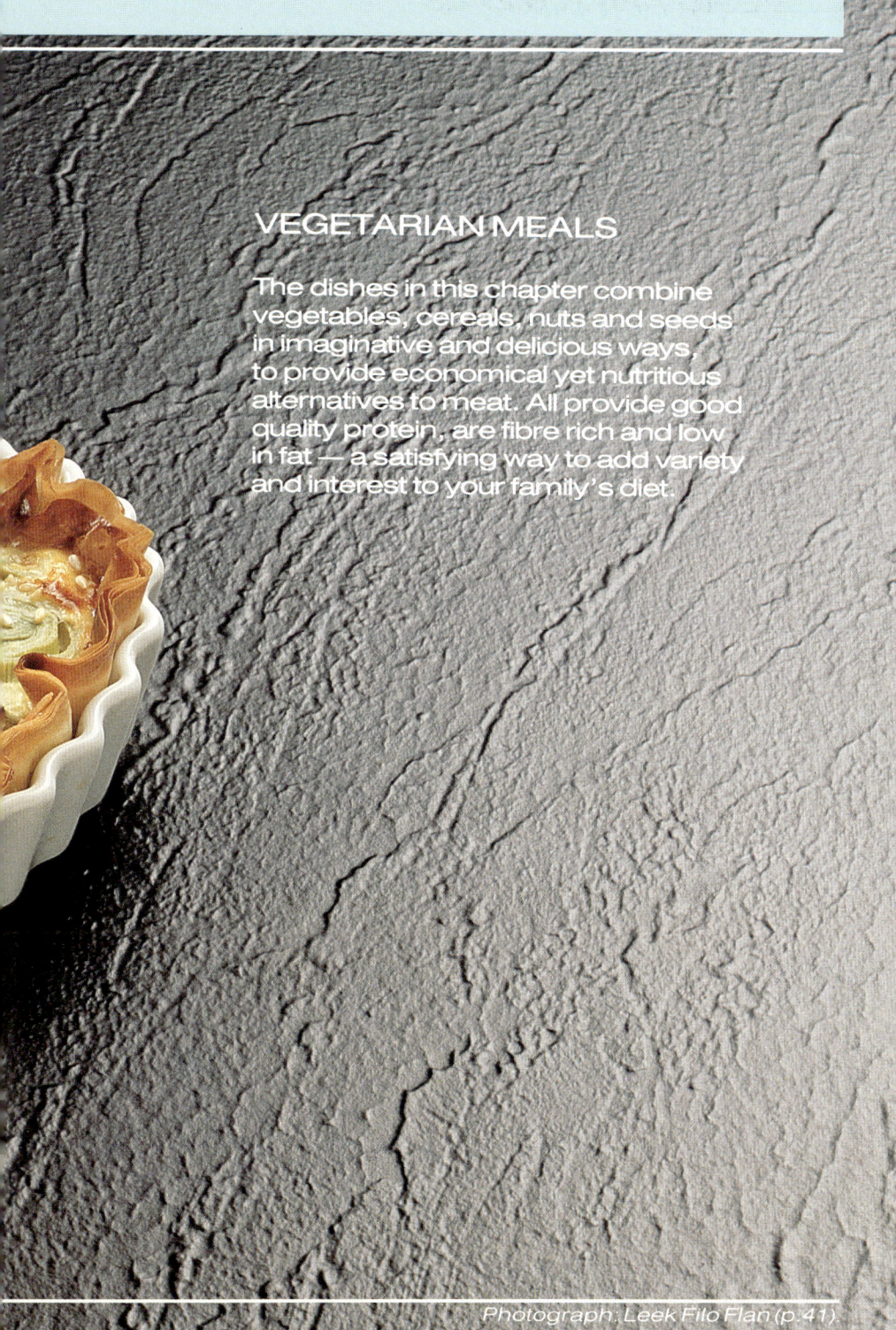

VEGETARIAN MEALS

The dishes in this chapter combine vegetables, cereals, nuts and seeds in imaginative and delicious ways, to provide economical yet nutritious alternatives to meat. All provide good quality protein, are fibre rich and low in fat — a satisfying way to add variety and interest to your family's diet.

Photograph: Leek Filo Flan (p.41).

BROCCOLI STACKS

Many people tend to think of pancakes as a sweet rather than a main course. By using non-fat milk in the sauce and only a small amount of cheese, this meal can be satisfying yet not too high in calories.

Pancakes

1 cup flour
1 egg
1 Tbsp polyunsaturated
   oil

1 ¼ cups non-fat milk
2 cups broccoli florets
4 tomatoes, sliced thinly

Sauce

1 Tbsp polyunsaturated
   oil
2 Tbsp flour
1 cup non-fat milk

1 Tbsp sunflower seeds
3 Tbsp grated
   parmesan cheese

Sift the flour and make a well in the centre. Add the egg, oil and half the milk. Blend to a paste. Add the remaining milk and blend to form a thin batter. Stand 1 hour. Heat a lightly greased non-stick frying pan. Pour in just enough batter to thinly cover the base. When set and light golden brown, turn and cook the second side. Repeat with remaining batter.

Sauce

Heat the oil in a saucepan. Add the flour and mix to a paste. Gradually add the milk. Heat and stir continuously for 3-4 minutes or until the sauce thickens. Add the sunflower seeds and parmesan cheese.

To Assemble The Stack

Steam the broccoli florets for 4-5 minutes or until tender but still slightly crunchy. Spread a pancake with sauce. Top this with broccoli florets and tomato slices. Place another pancake on top and repeat until the stack is 4-5 pancakes high. To reheat, cover with foil and bake at 180° C for 10-15 minutes.

Makes 2 stacks — four generous servings [1468 kJ (350 Cal) per serve].

Microwave

Make the pancakes as instructed.
In a microwave proof bowl blend the oil, flour,
parmesan cheese and sunflower seeds together.
Gradually add the milk, stirring until smooth.
Cook on 100% power for 3-4 minutes, stirring once
during cooking. Cover and cook the broccoli florets
on 100% power for 2-3 minutes or until tender.
Assemble as instructed. Cover and cook each
stack on 100% power for 2-3 minutes.

Photograph page 43

LEEK FILO FLAN

*A delicious low fat version of this very popular dish,
made without cream and high fat cheeses. Filo
pastry is paper thin and made with vegetable oil —
light in texture and full of flavour.*

4 sheets filo pastry
2 Tbsp polyunsaturated
  oil
3 cups finely sliced
  leeks
3 eggs
½ cup natural low fat
  yoghurt

½ cup non-fat milk
3 Tbsp grated
  parmesan cheese
freshly ground black
  pepper
1 tsp sesame seeds

Lay one sheet of filo pastry on a clean dry surface.
Brush sparingly with the oil. Cover with the second
sheet, brush with oil. Continue layering until all the
pastry is used. Use the layered pastry to line a 20
cm diameter quiche dish. Trim the pastry 2cm
above the level of the quiche dish. Fill with the
sliced leeks. Beat the eggs, yoghurt, milk and
parmesan cheese together. Pour into the quiche
dish. Sprinkle with the sesame seeds. Bake at
180°C for 40-45 minutes or until the egg is set.
Serves 5 [920 kJ (219 Cal) per serve].

Photograph page 38

VEGETABLE CURRY

Substantial and satisfying, this curry makes the most of whatever vegetables are in season — including some root vegetables. For a completely balanced meal, serve it with brown rice or wholegrain bread.

2 onions, finely chopped
1 clove garlic, peeled
    and finely chopped
1 Tbsp curry powder
½ cup water
⅓ cup peanuts
3 cups root vegetables
    peeled and sliced
    ie:- pumpkin, kumara,
    carrot and parsnip

3 cups green vegetables
    prepared into
    bite-sized pieces,
    ie:- green pepper,
    beans, peas, celery,
    courgettes, broccoli,
    cauliflower
½ cup water
2 Tbsp cornflour

Heat a large non-stick frying pan or wok. Add the onions, garlic, curry powder and first measure of water. Cook, stirring continuously until the onions are softened. Add the peanuts and root vegetables. Cook and stir for 10 minutes or until the vegetables soften. Add more water if necessary. Add the green vegetables, stir and toss for 4-5 minutes or until tender but still slightly crunchy. Mix the second measure of water and the cornflour together. Add to the vegetables. Cook for 2-3 minutes or until the juice thickens.
Serves 6 [403 kJ (86 Cal) per serve].

Variation: Try this curry served inside a cheese cracker pie crust (p.154).

Microwave
Place the onions, garlic, curry powder and first measure of water in a microwave proof dish. Cover and cook on 100% power for 2 minutes. Add the peanuts and root vegetables and cook on 100% power for 6-8 minutes. Add the green vegetables and cook on 100% power for 4-5 minutes or until softened. Reduce the second measure of water to 2 Tbsp and mix to a paste with the cornflour. Add to the vegetables and cook on 100% power for 2-3 minutes or until thickened. Stand for 3 minutes.

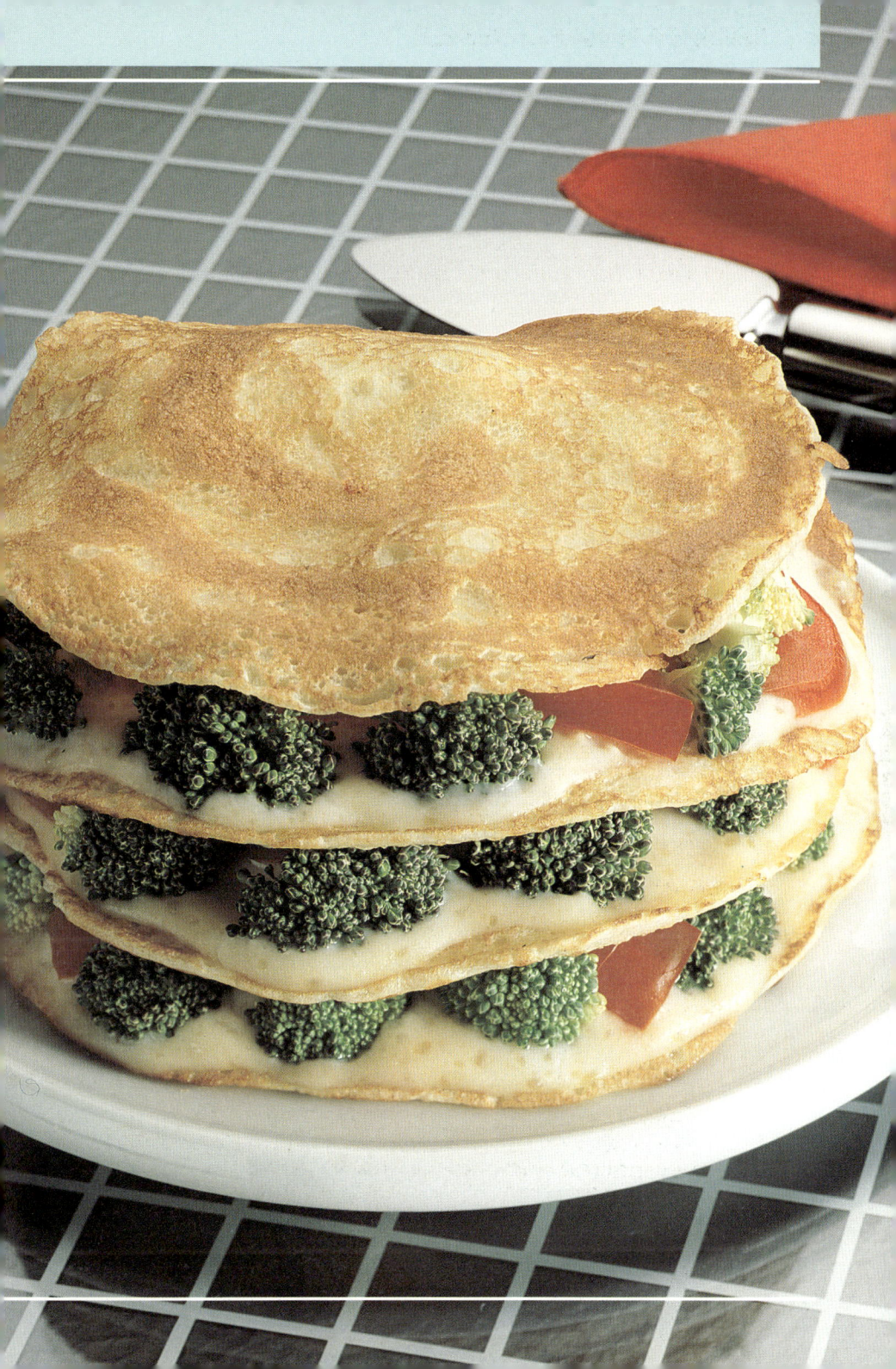

PASTA WITH STROGANOFF or ITALIAN SAUCE

A quick meal when you come home tired and hungry — full of vitamins, minerals and complex carbohydrate. Pasta is not fattening unless your sauce is laden with butter or cream. For extra fibre try wholemeal pasta varieties.

300 g dried pasta or 500 g fresh pasta
2-3 Tbsp grated parmesan cheese

Cook the pasta in boiling water until tender or according to the directions on the packet. Drain. Add the chosen sauce, mix well. Turn onto a serving platter and sprinkle with parmesan cheese. Serves 6 [Stroganoff 888 kJ (211 Cal) per serve] [Italian 782 (kJ (186 Cal) per serve].

Microwave
Bring a microwave proof bowl of water to the boil, add the pasta and cook until tender, or according to the directions on the packet. Drain.

Stroganoff Sauce
1 tsp polyunsaturated
  oil
1 onion, finely chopped
3 cups sliced
  mushrooms
2 Tbsp white wine

1 tsp finely chopped
  fresh marjoram or ½
  tsp dried marjoram
½ cup natural low fat
  yoghurt
freshly ground black
  pepper

Heat the oil in a saucepan and saute the onion for 2-3 minutes or until tender. Add the mushrooms, wine and marjoram. Simmer gently for 8-10 minutes. Stir in the yoghurt and season generously with pepper.

Microwave

Omit the oil. Cover and cook the onion on 100% power for 3 minutes. Add the mushrooms, wine and marjoram. Cook on 100% power for 3-4 minutes or until the mushrooms are soft. Mix 1 Tbsp cornflour and 1 Tbsp of water to a paste. Add to the sauce. Cook on 100% power for 2 minutes or until thickened. Stir in the yoghurt and pepper. Stand 5 minutes.

Italian Sauce

1 tsp polyunsaturated
 oil
2 cloves garlic, peeled
 and finely chopped
1 onion, finely chopped
500 g tomatoes,
 skinned and roughly
 chopped or 400 g tin
 whole peeled
 tomatoes, undrained

1 Tbsp finely chopped
 fresh thyme or 1 tsp
 dried thyme
2 Tbsp tomato paste
¼ cup water
freshly ground black
 pepper

Heat the oil in a saucepan. Saute the garlic and onion for 2-3 minutes or until tender. Add the tomatoes, thyme, tomato paste and water. Cover and simmer 10-15 minutes. Season generously with pepper.

Microwave

Omit the oil and water. Cover and cook the garlic and onions on 100% power for 3 minutes. Add the tomatoes, thyme and tomato paste. Cook on 100% power for 5-7 minutes. Stand 5 minutes.

Photograph page 175.

CHILLI BEAN NACHOS

Dried beans provide a nutritious alternative to meat. Protein-packed and fibre-filled, they are low in fat and contribute important vitamins and minerals for good health. This hot and spicy meal will be a favourite with the whole family.

¾ cup uncooked kidney beans
1 Tbsp polyunsaturated oil
1 onion, finely chopped
1 clove garlic, peeled and finely chopped
1 cup seasonal vegetables, finely diced eg:- carrot, celery, pepper

½ - 1 tsp chilli powder
400 g tin whole peeled tomatoes
2 Tbsp tomato puree
½ cup red wine
freshly ground black pepper
150 g corn chips
1 cup grated edam cheese
2 Tbsp finely chopped fresh parsley

Soak the beans in water overnight. Drain. Bring them to the boil in fresh water and simmer 45-50 minutes or until the beans are soft. Drain. Heat the oil and saute the onion and garlic for 2-3 minutes. Add the vegetables, beans and chilli powder. Saute another 2-3 minutes. Add the undrained tomatoes, tomato puree, red wine and pepper. Cover and simmer 20-30 minutes. Place the corn chips on an ovenproof serving platter. Top with the chilli bean mixture and cheese. Grill 5 minutes or until the cheese has melted. Sprinkle with parsley. Serve immediately.
Serves 6 [1586 kJ (378 Cal) per serve].

Variation: Use the chilli bean mixture as filling in taco shells with shredded lettuce, sliced tomato, grated edam cheese and grated carrot.

Note: A 310g tin of kidney beans may be substituted for the soaked and cooked beans. Drain and rinse thoroughly.

Microwave

Place the soaked beans in boiling water and cook on 100% power for 20 minutes. Stand 10 minutes. Drain. Omit the oil. Cover and cook the onion and garlic on 100% power for 2-3 minutes. Add the vegetables, beans, chilli powder, undrained tomatoes, tomato puree, red wine and pepper. Cook on 100% power for 10-12 minutes. Assemble nachos as instructed. Cook on 70% power for 3-4 minutes or until the cheese melts.

PIZZA

For a meal in a hurry, which is satisfying yet nutritious, pizza is ideal. For a quick base use wholemeal pita bread — low in fat and high in fibre.

2 tomatoes, peeled and chopped
1 clove garlic, peeled and finely chopped
1 onion, finely chopped
1/4 tsp dried basil or 1 tsp finely chopped fresh basil
1 Tbsp tomato paste
1 large wholemeal pita bread or 6 pita popettes
1/3 cup unsweetened crushed pineapple
1/3 cup grated edam cheese
1 Tbsp grated parmesan cheese
freshly ground black pepper

Simmer the tomatoes, garlic, onion, basil and tomato paste for 8-10 minutes or until the onion is soft. Spread over the pita bread. Top with pineapple, edam cheese, parmesan cheese and pepper. Bake at 200°C for 12-15 minutes or until golden brown. Serves 2 [1394 kJ (332 Cal) per serve].

Microwave

Cover and cook the tomatoes, garlic, onion, basil and tomato paste on 100% power for 4-5 minutes. Assemble pizza and cook on 100% power for 2-4 minutes or until the cheese has melted.

STUFFED PEPPERS

Peppers, especially green ones, contain more vitamin C than oranges. The rice, dried fruit and sunflower seeds provide a well-balanced fibre-rich vegetarian meal.

½ cup brown rice
4 green or red peppers
1 onion, finely chopped
¼ cup sunflower seeds
¼ cup chopped dried
    fruit (eg apricots,
    dates)

½ tsp dried thyme
  or 1 tsp fresh thyme
1 egg
1 cup tomato juice

Place the rice in boiling water and simmer 25-35 minutes or until tender but still chewy. Drain. Cut the peppers in half lengthwise or leave whole, but slice the top off. Remove the seeds. Combine rice, onion, sunflower seeds, dried fruit, thyme and egg. Stuff the peppers. Place the peppers and tomato juice in a baking dish. Bake at 180°C for 30-40 minutes or until the peppers have softened. Serve hot.
Serves 4 as a main course [816 kJ (194 Cal) per serve], or 8 as an entree.

Microwave
Place the rice and 2 cups of boiling water in a microwave proof bowl. Cook on 100% power for 12-15 minutes or until the rice is tender. Stand 6 minutes. Drain. Cover and cook the stuffed peppers on 100% power for 8-10 minutes or until the peppers soften. Stand 4 minutes.

Photograph page 163

COURGETTE BOATS

The fairly bland flavour of courgettes combines well with cheese in this recipe. The breadcrumbs and dried fruit add extra flavour and fibre.

4 medium courgettes
¼ cup grated edam cheese
½ cup natural low fat cottage cheese
¼ cup grated carrot
¼ cup currants
½ cup fresh wholemeal breadcrumbs
½ tsp dry mustard
2 spring onions, finely sliced
freshly ground black pepper
1-2 Tbsp water

Slice the courgettes in half lengthwise. Scoop out the seeds and discard. Mix together the edam cheese, cottage cheese, carrot, currants, breadcrumbs, mustard, spring onions, pepper and enough water to bind. Spoon the filling into the courgettes. Bake at 180°C for 30-35 minutes or until the courgettes are tender.
Serves 4 [575 kJ (137 Cal) per serve].

Microwave
Cover and cook the empty courgettes shells on 100% power for 3 minutes. Cover and cook the stuffed courgettes on 100% power for 3.-4 minutes. Stand 2 minutes.

CARROT LOAF

A quick and economical way to make the most of this versatile vegetable. This loaf is light and tasty yet packed with fibre and vitamins (especially vitamin A).

½ cup natural low fat
   yoghurt
2 Tbsp whole seed
   mustard
3 eggs

¼ cup wholemeal flour
freshly ground black
   pepper
6 cups grated carrot

I strongly recommend lining bottom and sides of tin with paper.

Mix all the ingredients together. Turn into a greased 9cm x 16cm loaf tin. Cover with foil and bake at 180°C for 40-50 minutes or until the mixture is set. Stand 10 minutes before turning out. Serve hot or cold with natural yoghurt as a sauce.
Serves 6 [377 kJ (90 Cal) per serve].

Variation: Substitute 3 cups of grated carrot with 3 cups grated parsnip.

Microwave
Turn the mixture into a lined 20cm microwave proof ring mould. Elevate and cook on 100% power for 15-17 minutes or until dry to touch. Stand 5 minutes before turning out.

Photograph opposite page.

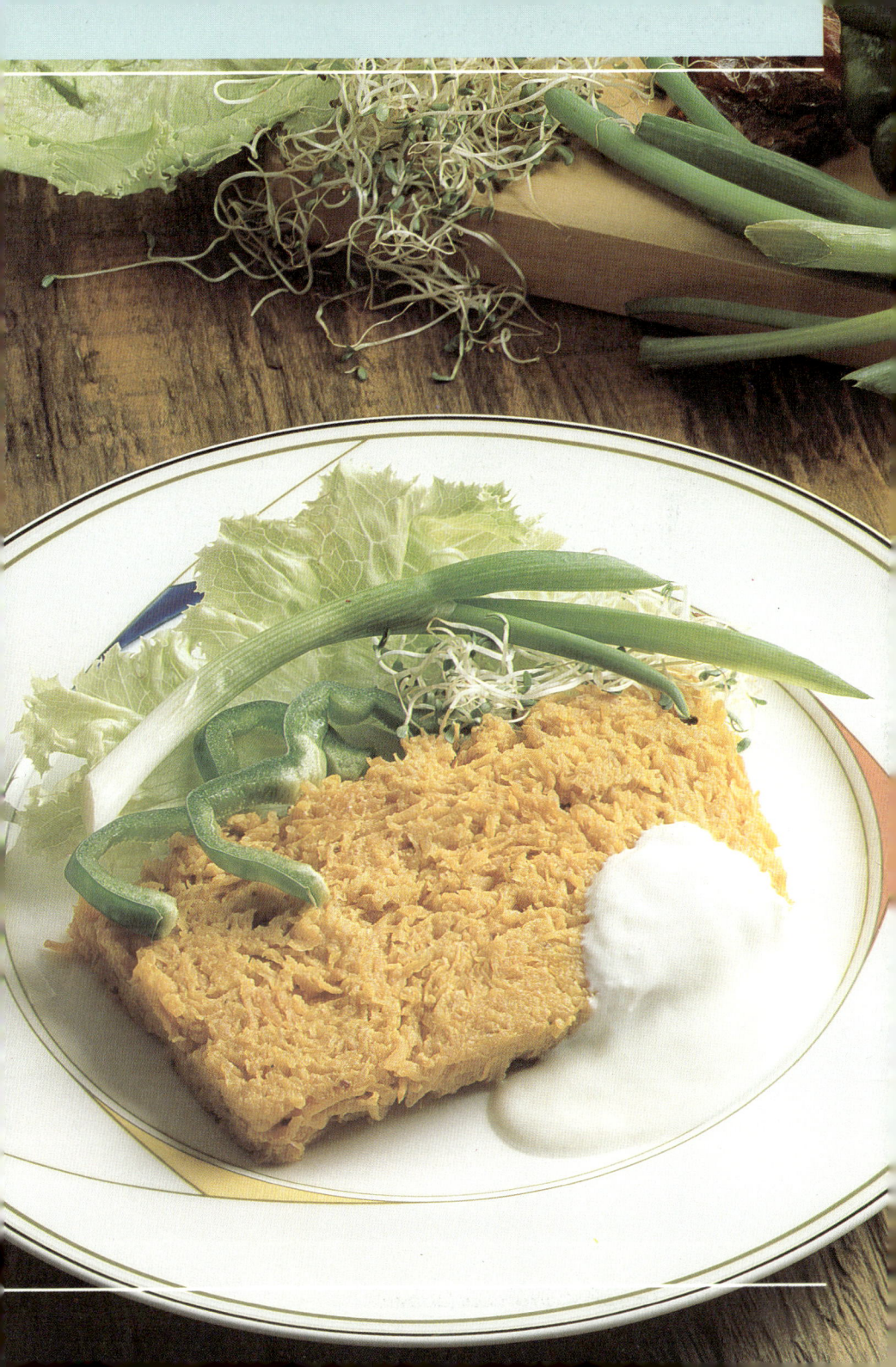

TOFU AND VEGETABLE TOSS

This high fibre rice and tofu dish is a meal on its own — a completely balanced low fat vegetarian meal. The mixture of tofu and rice is as nutritious as meat.

250 g tofu (bean curd)
3 Tbsp soy sauce
1 cup brown rice
1 Tbsp polyunsaturated
  oil
1 onion, finely chopped
1 clove garlic, peeled
  and finely chopped

½-1 tsp ground
  coriander
1 carrot, finely sliced
1 apple, cored and
  sliced
½ cup water
4-5 spinach leaves,
  roughly chopped

Cut the tofu into bite-sized pieces and marinate in soy sauce overnight. Cook the rice in boiling water for 30-40 minutes or until tender. Drain. Heat the oil in a large heavy based saucepan and saute the onion, garlic and coriander for 2-3 minutes or until the onion softens. Add the carrot, apple and water. Cover and simmer for 10 minutes. Carefully stir in the tofu, soy sauce and rice. Heat for 3-4 minutes. Stir in the spinach, taking care not to break up the tofu. Serve immediately.
Serves 4 [1041 kJ (248 Cal) per serve].

Microwave
Place the rice and 3 cups boiling water in a large microwave proof bowl. Cook on 100% power for 20 minutes. Stand 10 minutes. Drain. Omit the oil and reduce the water to ¼ cup. Cover and cook the onion, garlic and coriander on 100% power for 2-3 minutes. Add the carrots and cook on 100% power for 4 minutes. Carefully stir in the tofu, soy sauce, apple, water and rice. Cook on 100% power for 6-8 minutes or until the carrots are tender. Stir in the spinach. Stand 4 minutes. Serve immediately.

QUICK CORN QUICHE

This quiche makes its own base — a novel idea when time is limited.

450 g tin whole kernel
    corn, drained
3 medium tomatoes,
    sliced
½ cup pancake mix
1 cup non-fat milk

2 eggs
1 Tbsp grated
    parmesan cheese
freshly ground black
    pepper
1 Tbsp grated
    parmesan cheese

Place the corn and tomatoes in a 20cm diameter ceramic quiche dish. Beat the pancake mix, milk, eggs, first measure of parmesan cheese and pepper together. Pour over the corn and tomatoes. Sprinkle with the second measure of parmesan cheese. Bake at 200° C for 25-30 minutes or until set and golden brown.
Serves 5 [913 kJ (217 Cal) per serve].

Variation: Replace the corn and tomato with:-

1 cup cooked, drained
    and chopped
    spinach

1 cup sliced
    mushrooms

STUFFED POTATOES

Potatoes can make a marvellous meal — and when eaten in moderation are not fattening. Potatoes baked in their jackets have better flavour and food value. They rate well in the fibre stakes and although they are good sources of vitamins and minerals, potatoes are not high in calories.

4 medium potatoes

Corn Filling

½ cup non-fat milk
½ cup whole kernel
  corn
½ cup chopped, red or
  green pepper

1 Tbsp grated
  parmesan cheese
freshly ground black
  pepper
1 Tbsp grated
  parmesan cheese

Bean Filling

315 g tin four bean mix
3 Tbsp finely chopped
  fresh parsley
½ cup natural low fat
  yoghurt

¼ cup non-fat milk
freshly ground black
  pepper

Pumpkin Filling

1 cup cooked pumpkin
  puree
½ cup natural low fat
  yoghurt

¼ tsp ground cloves
2 spring onions, finely
  sliced

Wash and scrub the potatoes. Pierce and bake at 180°C for 45-60 minutes or until softened. Cut the potatoes in half, scoop out the cooked potato, leaving the skin halves intact. Refill with chosen filling. Reheat at 180°C for 10 minutes.
Serves 4 [Corn 629 kJ (150 Cal) per serve],
[Bean 806 kJ (192 Cal) per serve],
[Pumpkin 465 kJ (111 Cal) per serve].

Corn Filling

Mix the cooked potato, milk, corn, red or green pepper, the first measure of parmesan cheese and black pepper together. Fill the potato halves, sprinkle with the second measure of parmesan cheese.

Bean Filling

Rinse and drain the beans. Mix the cooked potato, beans, parsley, yoghurt, milk and pepper together.

Pumpkin Filling

Mix the cooked potato, pumpkin, yoghurt, cloves and spring onions together.

Microwave

Cook on 100% power for 10-12 minutes or until softened. Stand 4 minutes. Cook stuffed potatoes on 100% power for 2-3 minutes.

Photograph page 163

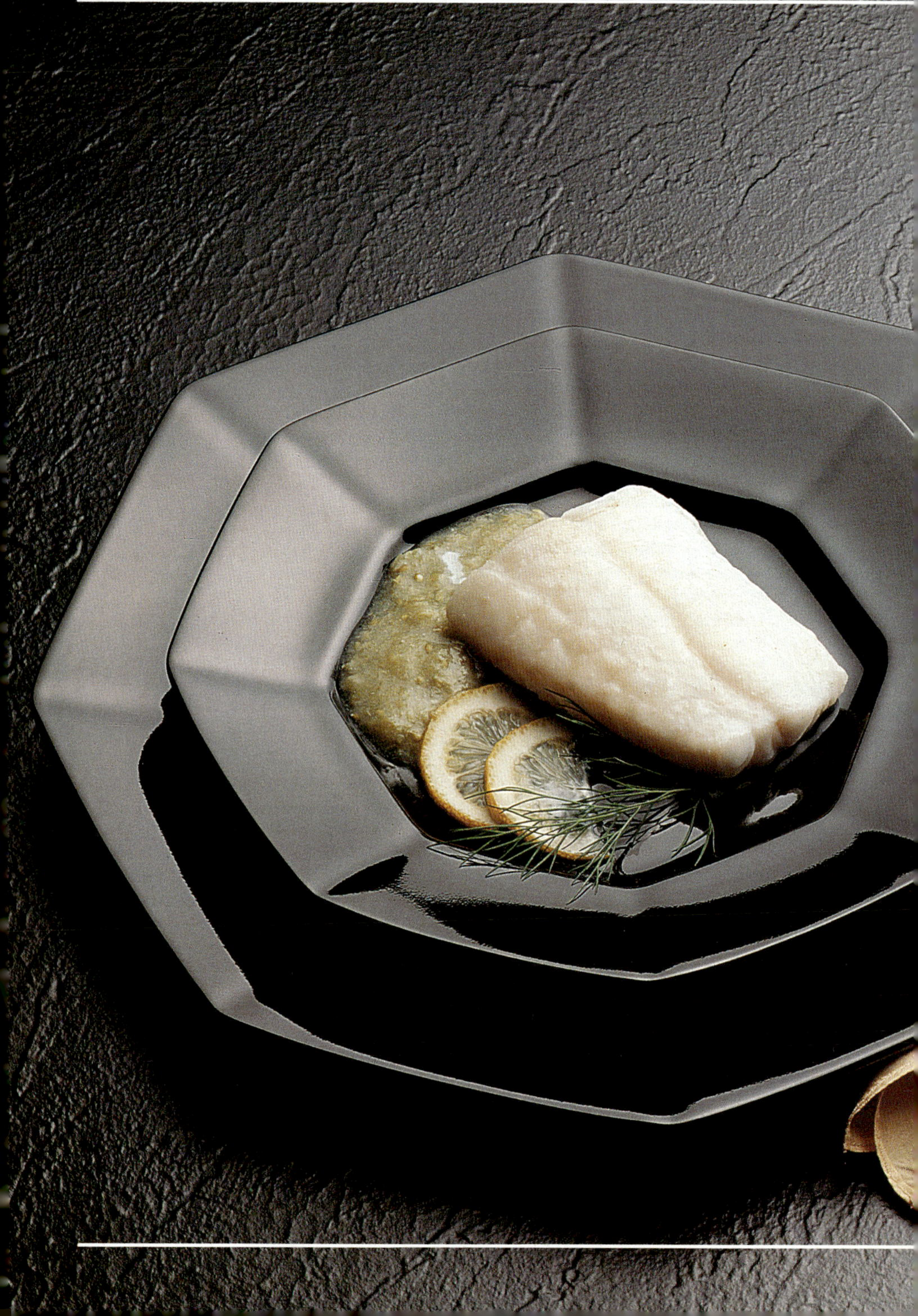

FISH

Fish being high in protein and low in fat is a delicious and nutritious alternative to meat and chicken. It should however be handled with care, cooked quickly so that it doesn't dry out, and served with light sauces and accompaniments that enhance its delicate flavour. The recipes that follow use fish in a variety of imaginative and innovative ways, sure to please the whole family.

Photograph: Fish Fillets with Gooseberry Sauce (p.58).

FISH FILLETS WITH GOOSEBERRY SAUCE

The tang of the sauce suits the mildness of the fish. The fibre-rich gooseberries complement the smooth textured fillets.

3 cups fresh or frozen
   gooseberries
¼ cup water

1 Tbsp sugar
600 g fish fillets
   eg. orange roughy

Top and tail the gooseberries. Place the gooseberries, water and sugar in a saucepan and simmer gently for 10-15 minutes or until the gooseberries are tender. Puree. Keep warm. Grill the fish for 2-3 minutes each side or until the fish is white and flakes easily with a fork. Pour the sauce over the fish. Serve immediately.
Serves 6 [594 kJ (141 Cal) per serve].

Microwave
Omit the water. Cover and cook the gooseberries and sugar on 100% power, for 4-5 minutes if fresh, or 6-7 minutes if frozen. Puree. Keep warm. Cover and cook the fish on 70% power for 6-8 minutes or until the fish is white and flakes easily with a fork. Stand 3 minutes.

Photograph page 56

MARINATED FISH SALAD

Fish does not lose much value in cooking, so the main advantage in this recipe is the flavour, plus the generous amount of vitamin C in the citrus juice.

500 g fish fillets eg. ling
½ cup lemon juice
1 onion, finely chopped
2 bay leaves
freshly ground black
   pepper

1 cup peeled and
   cubed cucumber
½ cup chopped green
   pepper
½ cup natural low fat
   yoghurt

Cut the fish into bite-sized pieces. Mix together the fish, lemon juice, onion, bay leaves and pepper in a non-metallic bowl. Refrigerate and marinate for several hours or until the fish is white throughout. Discard the marinade and bay leaves. Combine the fish, onion, cucumber, green pepper and yoghurt. Mix well and serve chilled.
Serves 4 [711 kJ (169 Cal) per serve].

FISH RATATOUILLE

A taste of the Mediterranean, but not too high in fat. The green vegetables add fibre and plenty of vitamin C.

3 cups unpeeled, chopped eggplant
1 tsp salt
1 onion, chopped into wedges
1 clove garlic, peeled and finely chopped

2 courgettes, sliced
1 green pepper, sliced
400 g tin whole peeled tomatoes
2 Tbsp tomato paste
400 g lemon fish fillets

Sprinkle the egg plant with the salt and stand for one hour. Wash thoroughly in cold running water. Drain. Heat a non-stick frying pan and saute the onion and garlic for 2-3 minutes or until softened. And the eggplant, courgette, pepper, undrained tomatoes and tomato paste. Cover and simmer for 30-35 minutes or until the vegetables soften. Cut the fish into bite-sized pieces and add to the vegetables. Simmer 5 minutes. Serve immediately.
Serves 5 [645 kJ (154 Cal) per serve].

Microwave
Cook the onion and garlic in a microwave proof dish on 100% power for 3 minutes. Add the eggplant, courgettes, pepper, undrained tomatoes and tomato paste. Cover and cook on 100% power for 15-17 minutes or until the vegetables soften. Add the fish and stand 8 minutes. Cook on 100% power for 2 minutes.

FISH CAKES

Patties do not have to be fried — grill or bake instead to keep the fat content low.

3 cups cold cooked
   mashed potato
200 g tin tuna, packed
   in brine
1 Tbsp lemon juice
2 spring onions, finely
   chopped
2 Tbsp finely chopped
   fresh parsley

½ cup natural low fat
   cottage cheese
1 egg white
freshly ground black
   pepper
1 cup fresh wholemeal
   breadcrumbs
¼ cup sesame seeds
¼ cup non-fat milk

Combine the potato, drained tuna, lemon juice, spring onions, parsley, cottage cheese, egg white and pepper. Take spoonfuls of the mixture and shape into round cakes. Mix the breadcrumbs and sesame seeds together. Dip the fish cakes in milk and coat with the breadcrumb mixture. Refrigerate for 2 hours before cooking. Bake at 180°C for 30 minutes or fry in a lightly greased non-stick frying pan for 6-8 minutes or until golden brown. Serve with tomato sauce (p 18).
Serves 6 [1141 kJ (272 Cal) per serve].

Variation: This recipe works equally well with other types of tinned fish.

FLORENTINE FISH

An attractive and different way to serve fish, which retains its low fat content and ensures its delicate flavour is not overpowered. The spinach and mushrooms add fibre and vitamins for good health.

½ cup cooked and
   chopped spinach
1 cup finely chopped
   mushrooms
2 Tbsp natural low fat
   yoghurt

freshly ground black
   pepper
4 fish fillets
   eg. lemonfish, terakihi
2 Tbsp lemon juice

Mix the spinach, mushrooms, yoghurt and pepper together. Trim the fillets and roll into 4 hollow tubes, secure with toothpicks. Place upright in a baking dish and fill each tube with the spinach mixture. Place any extra filling around the tubes. Sprinkle with the lemon juice. Cover and bake at 180°C for 15-20 minutes or until the fish is white and flakes easily with a fork.
Serves 4 [628 kJ (150 Cal) per serve].

Microwave
Cover and cook on 70% power for 5-7 minutes or until the fish is white. Stand 3 minutes.

FLOUNDER WITH CUCUMBER

Rather than the traditional lemon wedges try cucumber as a refreshing accompaniment to fish — cool and crisp, yet still low in fat.

4 flounder, cleaned
½ cup non-fat milk
½ cup wholemeal
  flour
freshly ground black
  pepper

1 Tbsp polyunsaturated
  oil
1½ cups cucumber
  chunks, peeled and
  deseeded
lemon wedges for
  garnish

Dip each flounder in milk, then in wholemeal flour seasoned with pepper. Heat the oil in a non-stick frying pan. Fry each flounder for 6 - 8 minutes on each side or until golden brown. Remove from pan and keep warm. Add the cucumber chunks to the pan and stir until golden brown. Serve the flounder and cucumber garnished with lemon wedges.
Serves 4 [1012 kJ (241 Cal) per serve].

Variation: For a special occasion use a melon baller to make cucumber balls. Cook as directed for chunks.

FISH PARCELS

A novel idea for baking fish — easy to prepare, quick and fun to serve. The parcels can't be microwaved but follow the microwave instructions for an equally tasty alternative.

1 Tbsp polyunsaturated oil
4 fish fillets eg. terakihi, cod
1 cup finely cut carrot sticks

1 cup finely cut celery sticks
1 cup sliced mushrooms
freshly ground black pepper
2 Tbsp lemon juice

Cut four greaseproof paper circles of 35cm diameter. Brush sparingly with the oil. Trim the fish fillets into two equal halves. Lay half a fillet on the lower half of each circle. Place one quarter of the carrot, celery and mushrooms on the fillet and top with the second half of the fillet. Season generously with pepper and sprinkle with lemon juice. Fold the free half of the paper over the fish to form a parcel. Twist and fold the edges together to form an airtight seal. Place on a baking tray so they do not touch each other. Bake at 180°C for 15 minutes or until the parcels are puffed up. Serve immediately. Each diner unwraps their own parcel.
Serves 4 [659 kJ (157 Cal) per serve].

Variation: Wrap in foil and bake or barbeque as instructed.

Microwave
Omit paper wrapping. Place fish in microwave proof dish. Cover with plastic film and cook on 70% power for 6-8 minutes. Stand 3 minutes.

Photograph opposite page

Photograph: Fish Parcels (above).

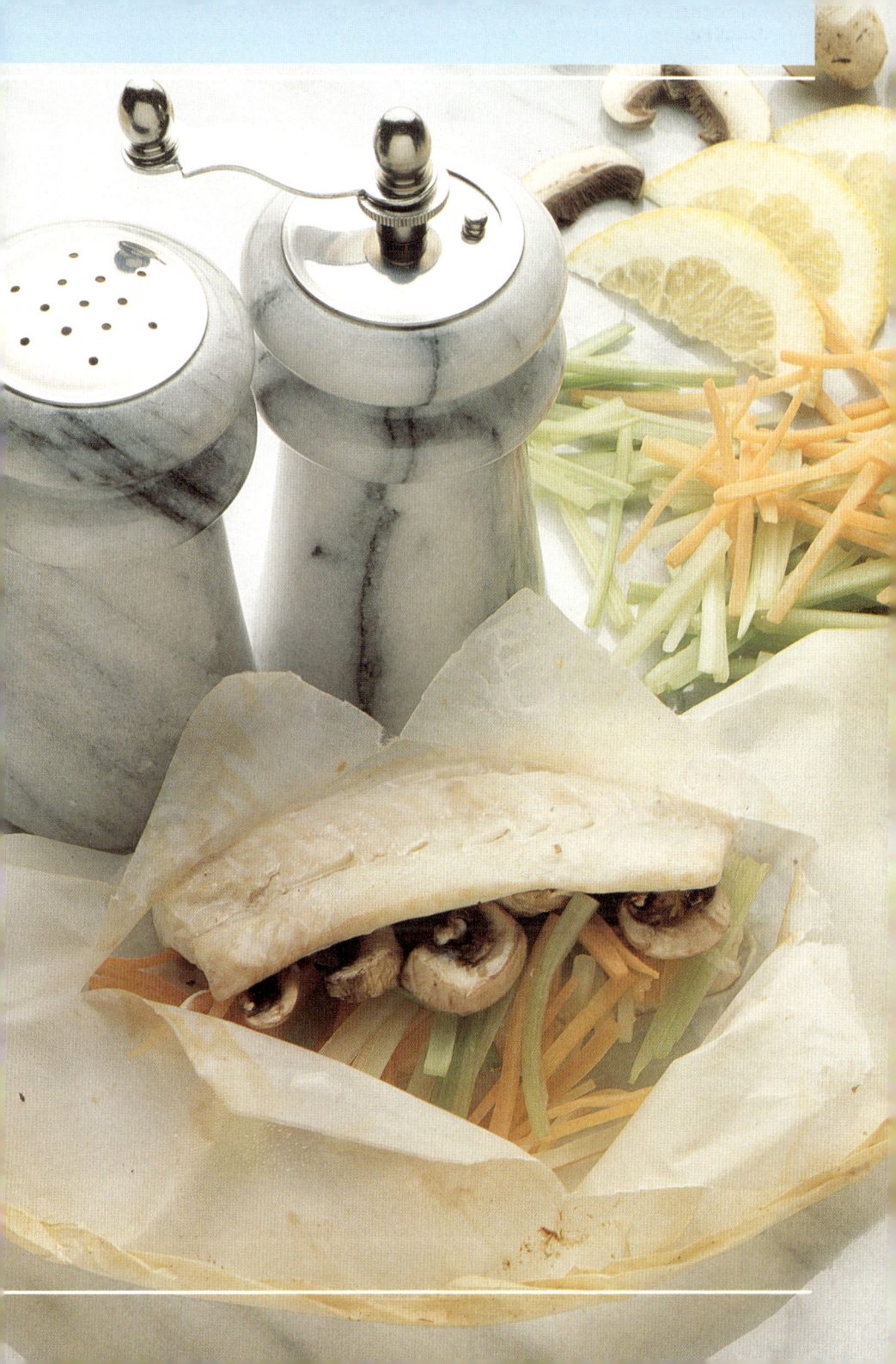

PLAITED FISH

An excellent dinner party idea — looks impressive yet is quite simple to prepare. The light wine sauce will not overpower the delicate flavour of fish nor add too many calories.

4 fish fillets eg. terakihi, snapper
1 cup white wine
3-4 bay leaves
1 onion, finely chopped
2 tsp cornflour

2 tsp water
1 tsp sugar
freshly ground black pepper
fresh dill for garnish

Select even sized fillets. Trim the fillets to give twelve strips of even width. Take three strips and plait together. Tuck ends under. Repeat with remaining strips. Transfer into a roasting dish. Add the wine, bay leaves and onion. Cover and bake at 180°C for 10-15 minutes or until the fish is white and tender. Remove the fish and keep warm. Strain the cooking juices into a small saucepan. Mix the cornflour and water to a paste, add to the cooking juices and heat gently for 2-3 minutes or until thickened. Add the sugar and season generously with pepper. Serve the plaits and sauce garnished with fresh dill.
Serves 4 [810 kJ (193 Cal) per serve].

Microwave
Cover and cook on 70% power for 5-7 minutes or until the fish is white and tender. Stand 3 minutes. Prepare the sauce as instructed. Cook on 100% power for 2-3 minutes.

Photograph page 166

BAKED WHOLE FISH

The ginger adds extra flavour to this dish and gives it an oriental mood. Balance this mainly protein dish with brown rice or baked potatoes and green vegetables, to provide fibre and complementary flavours.

1.5 kg whole fish
  eg. cod, snapper
¼ cup lemon juice
½ cup white wine
2 tsp brown sugar
1 tsp finely chopped
  root ginger

1 clove garlic, peeled
  and finely chopped
freshly ground black
  pepper
lemon wedges for
  garnish

Clean the fish and remove the scales. Wash and dry the gut cavity. Leave head and tail intact or remove if wished. Place the fish in a baking dish. Mix together the lemon juice, wine, brown sugar, ginger, garlic and pepper, pour over the fish. Bake covered at 180°C for 30-40 minutes, or until the fish flakes easily with a fork. Baste occasionally during cooking. Serve hot or chilled. Garnish with lemon wedges.
Serves 4 [504 kJ (120 Cal) per serve].

Microwave
Reduce the wine to ¼ cup. Cover and cook on 70% power for 12-14 minutes or until the fish flakes easily with a fork. Stand 5 minutes.

Barbeque
Reduce the wine to ¼ cup. Wrap the fish in foil and cook on a barbeque for 30-40 minutes or until the fish flakes easily with a fork.
Turn frequently during cooking.

MUSSELS AND PASTA

Shellfish are particularly rich in minerals, especially iron and zinc. They are low in fat and not as high in cholesterol as once thought.

1 dozen fresh mussels
500 g fresh fettucine or
   300 g dried kluski
   pasta
½ cup natural low fat
   yoghurt

1 Tbsp finely chopped
   fresh dill
1 Tbsp finely chopped
   orange rind
freshly ground black
   pepper

Steam the mussels for 5-10 minutes or until the shells open. Remove from shells. Keep warm. Cook the pasta according to the directions on the packet. Drain. Toss the pasta, mussels, yoghurt, dill, orange rind and pepper together. Serve immediately.
Serves 5 [736 kJ (175 Cal) per serve].

Note: Canned or frozen mussels may be substituted for the fresh mussels. Heat before adding to the pasta

Microwave
Cook the mussels on 100% power for 6-7 minutes or until the shells open. Bring a large bowl of water to the boil, add the pasta and cook according to the directions on the packet.

Photograph opposite page

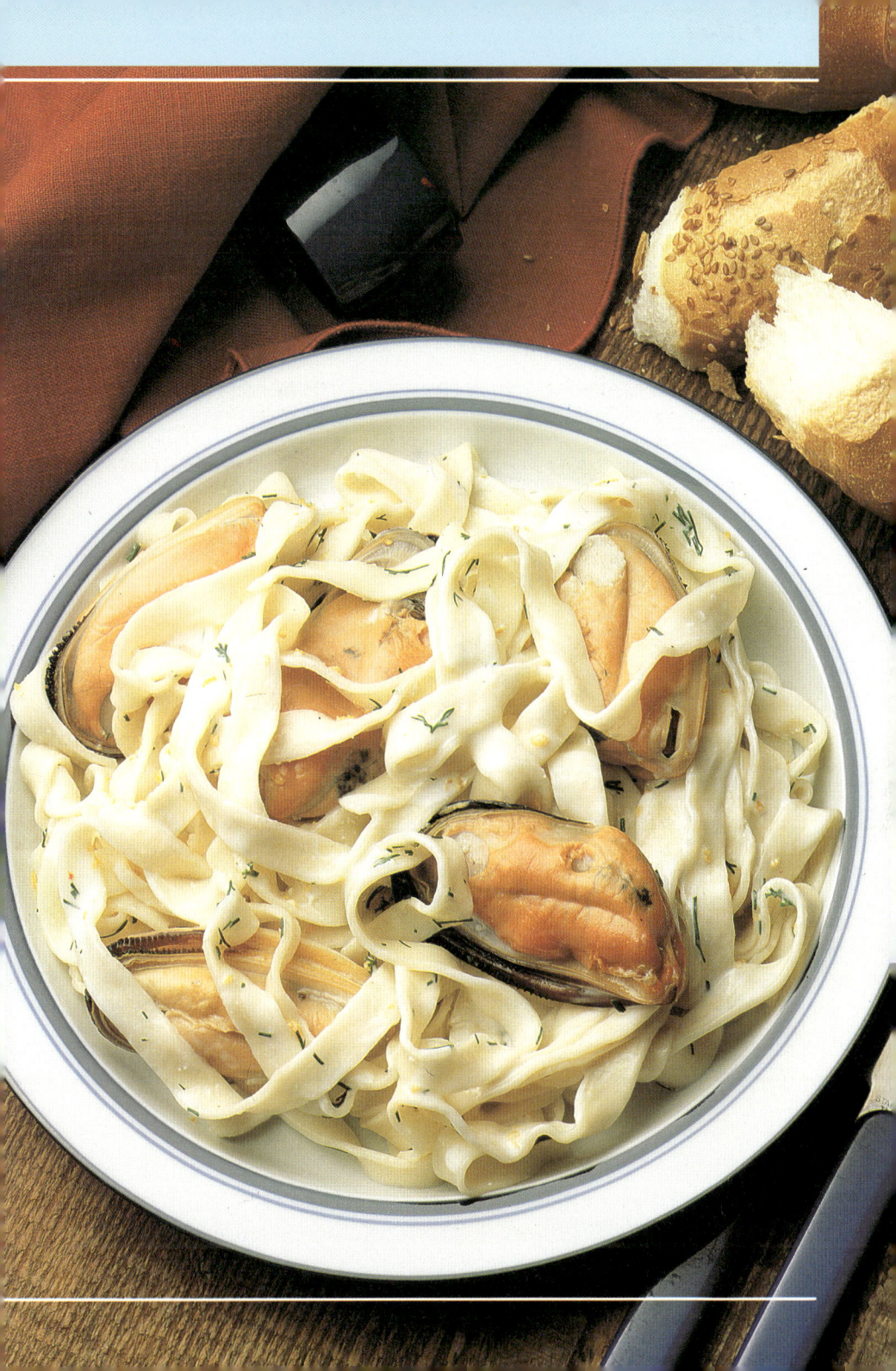

SMOKED HOKI PIE

This fish pie is a popular family meal. Calories are kept low by using non-fat milk. For a balanced meal serve it with plenty of fresh vegetables, adding fibre and vitamins.

1 Tbsp polyunsaturated oil
1 onion, finely chopped
1 Tbsp flour
1 cup non-fat milk
400 g smoked hoki fillet
½ cup finely chopped celery
2 medium potatoes, peeled and sliced thinly

Heat the oil in a heavy based saucepan. Add the onion and saute 2-3 minutes or until softened. Remove from the heat, add the flour and mix well. Gradually add the milk. Return to the heat and stir as the sauce thickens. Reserve ¾ cup of the sauce. Remove the skin and cut the hoki into bite-sized pieces. Mix the hoki, celery and sauce together. Turn into a casserole dish. Layer the potato slices and reserved sauce on top of the hoki mixture. Bake at 190° C for 30-40 minutes or until the potatoes are softened and golden brown.
Serves 5 [893 kJ (213 Cal) per serve].

Microwave

Cover and cook the potatoes on 100% power for 8 minutes. Cover and cook the oil and onion on 100% power for 3 minutes. Blend in the flour and milk. Cook on 100% power for 3-4 minutes, stirring once during cooking. Turn the fish mixture into a microwave proof dish. Top with the cooked potatoes and remaining sauce. Cover and cook on 70% power for 3-4 minutes. Stand 5 minutes. Grill to brown if wished.

FISH SOUFFLE

A light, appetising dish that can be made when unexpected guests arrive for dinner as most ingredients are usually in the pantry. Drain the fish well as tinned products are often high in salt.

3 eggs
1 Tbsp polyunsaturated
 oil
2 Tbsp flour
1 cup non-fat milk
200 g tin tuna, packed
 in brine
2 Tbsp lemon juice

2 spring onions, finely
 chopped
2 Tbsp grated
 parmesan cheese
freshly ground black
 pepper
1 Tbsp grated
 parmesan cheese

Separate the eggs. Heat the oil in a small saucepan. Add the flour and blend well. Gradually add the milk and stir as the sauce thickens. Stir in the egg yolks, drained tuna, lemon juice, spring onions, first measure of parmesan cheese and pepper. Beat the egg whites until stiff. Fold into the fish mixture. Turn into a lightly greased 18cm diameter souffle dish. Sprinkle with the second measure of parmesan cheese and bake at 180°C for 45-50 minutes or until golden brown and the mixture is set. Serve immediately. Alternatively turn into 6 individual ramekin dishes and bake 8-12 minutes or until the mixture is set.
Serves 6 [715 kJ (170 Cal) per serve].

Note: The mixture may be frozen before it is cooked. Do not thaw, cook from frozen at 180°C allowing 1-1¼ hours for the large, or 16-18 minutes for the small.

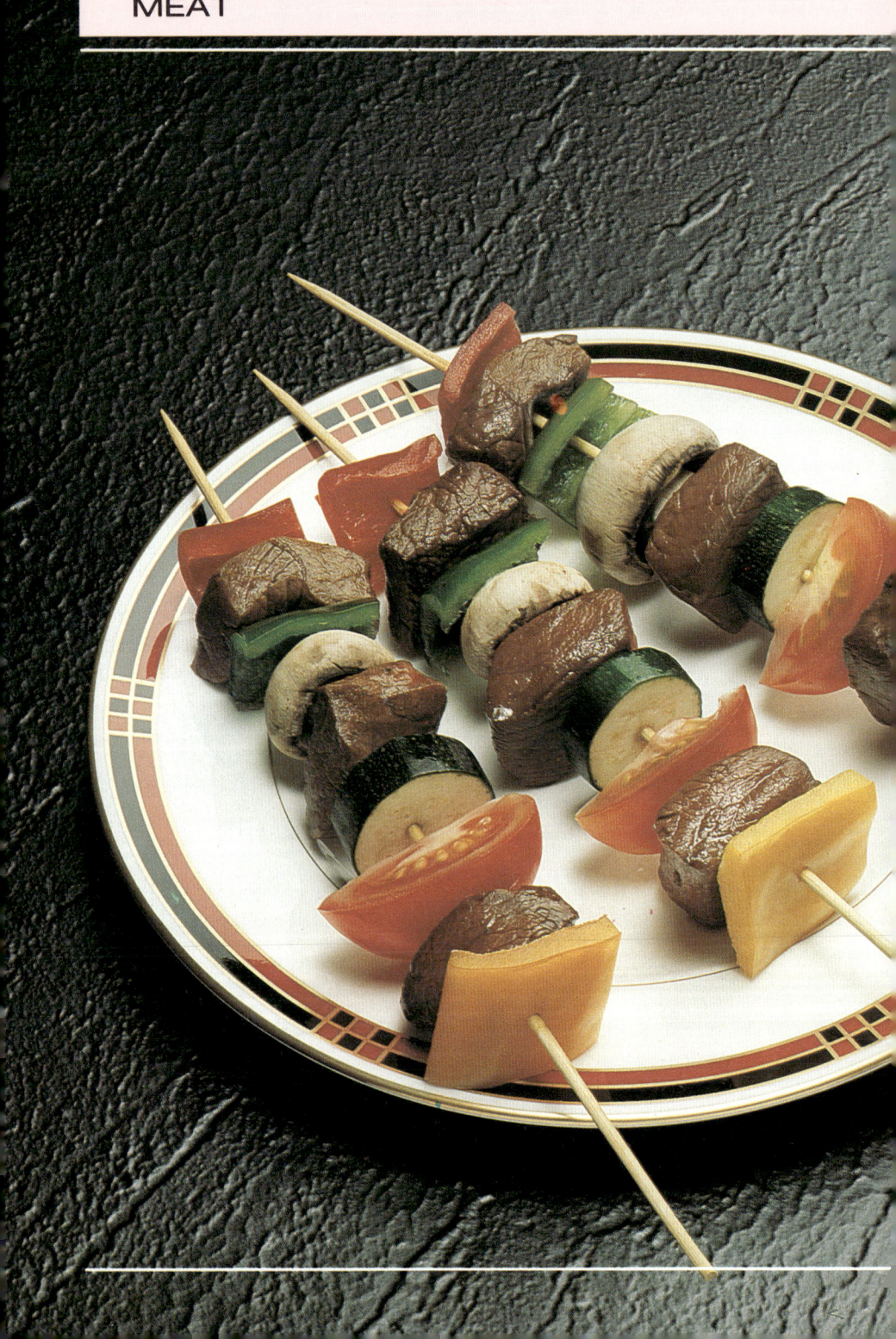

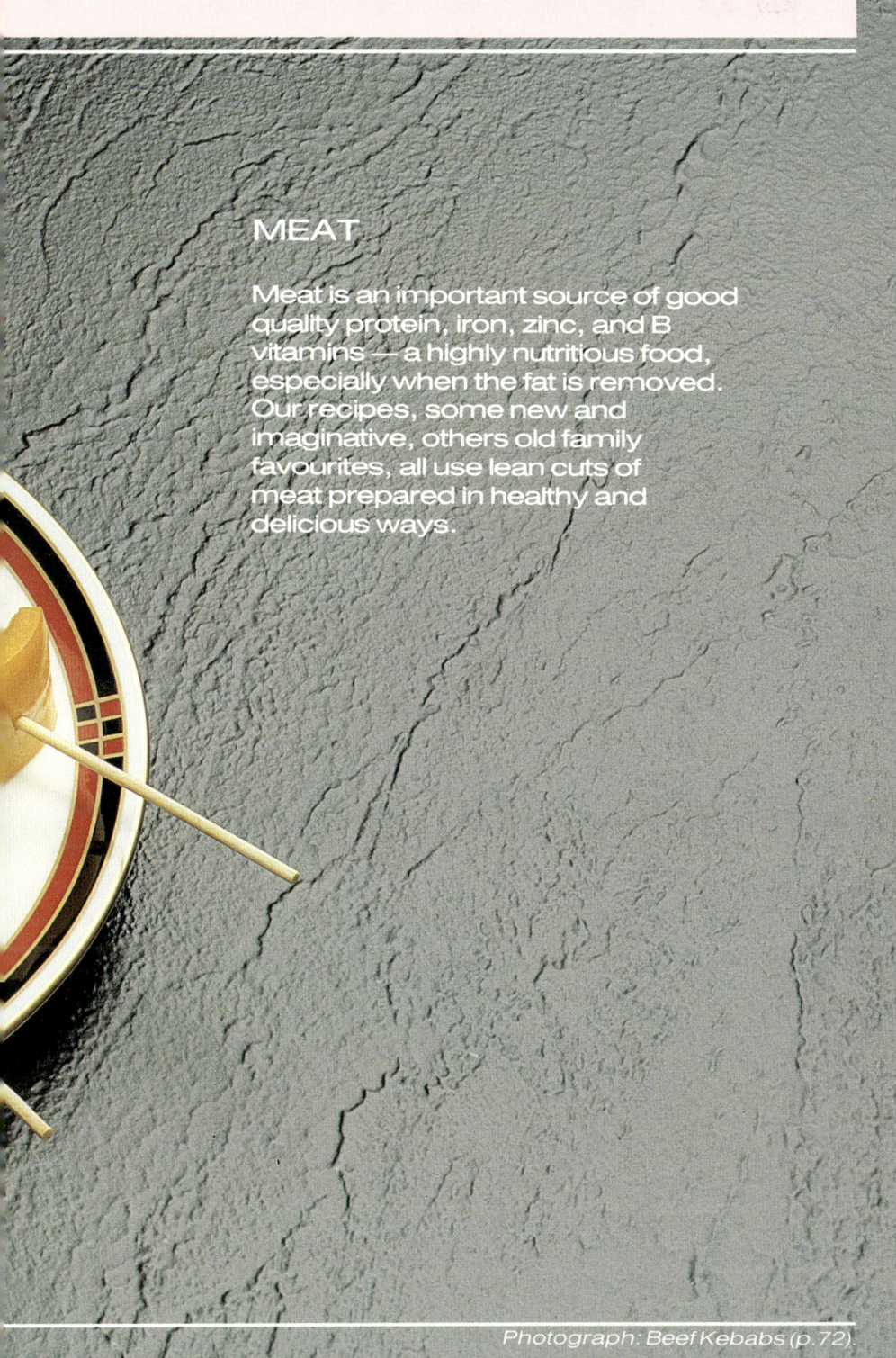

MEAT

Meat is an important source of good quality protein, iron, zinc, and B vitamins — a highly nutritious food, especially when the fat is removed. Our recipes, some new and imaginative, others old family favourites, all use lean cuts of meat prepared in healthy and delicious ways.

Photograph: Beef Kebabs (p. 72).

BEEF KEBABS

Kebabs make one of the best and most enjoyable ways of presenting really lean meat, while also making it go a long way. The marinade increases tenderness, flavour and shortens cooking time.

400 g lean blade steak
1 clove garlic, peeled
   and finely chopped
2 Tbsp soy sauce
2 Tbsp water
1 Tbsp Worcestershire
   sauce

4 cups seasonal
   vegetables, cut into
   bite-sized pieces
   eg: tomatoes,
   mushrooms, red and
   green peppers,
   green and yellow
   courgettes, onions.

Remove all visible fat from the meat and cut into 2cm cubes. Mix the meat, garlic, soy sauce, water and Worcestershire sauce together. Marinate 1-2 hours. Thread the meat and vegetables onto kebab sticks. Grill or barbeque for 10-15 minutes, turning frequently until the meat is brown and tender.
Serves 4 [798 kJ (190 Cal) per serve].

Photograph page 70

BEEF STIR-FRY

To retain the colour, texture and food value of this dish, quick cooking is essential. Serve with brown rice or baked potatoes for a well-balanced meal.

500 g lean beef
   schnitzel
1 clove garlic, peeled
   and finely chopped
2 Tbsp soy sauce
1 cup broccoli florets
425 g tin baby corn,
   drained

2 carrots, finely sliced
230 g tin water
   chestnuts, drained
   (optional)
¼ cup water
1 tsp cornflour

Remove all visible fat from the meat and cut into 2cm wide strips. Combine the meat, garlic and soy saucé and marinate for 1 hour. Saute for 3-4 minutes in a non-stick frying pan or a lightly oiled wok. Add the broccoli, baby corn, carrots and water chestnuts. Stir-fry for 4-6 minutes or until the vegetables are tender but still slightly crisp. Mix the water and cornflour together. Add to the frying pan, stir and heat 1-2 minutes or until thickened. Serve immediately.
Serves 4 [1113 kJ (265 Cal) per serve].

MUSTARD STEAKS

The secret for success with this recipe is being well organised before you start cooking. Replacing the usual cream with yoghurt in the sauce helps to keep the fat content down.

4 lean fillet steaks
3 Tbsp brandy
½ cup water
1 Tbsp whole seed
    mustard

¼ cup natural low fat
    yoghurt
freshly ground black
    pepper

Remove all visible fat from the meat. Heat a frying pan until very hot. Dry fry the steaks for 2-3 minutes each side or until cooked to your preference. Remove from the pan and keep warm. Take the pan off the heat and add the brandy, water and mustard. Stir well. Stir in the yoghurt and season with pepper. Return the steaks to the pan and coat with the sauce. Serve immediately.
Serves 4 [861 kJ (205 Cal) per serve].

LAMB CURRY

This curry has a deep mellow flavour that's not too hot. Serve it with the traditional side dishes for contrasting textures and flavours — and to make a completely balanced meal.

700 g lean lamb —
    forequarter or
    shoulder
1 onion, finely chopped
1 clove garlic, peeled
    and finely chopped

1 Tbsp curry powder
2 Tbsp tomato paste
½ tsp finely chopped
    chillis or ¼ tsp chilli
    powder
1½ cups water

Remove all visible fat from the meat and cut into 2cm cubes. Brown the meat in a non-stick saucepan. (It is easier to brown a few pieces at a time than all at once). Place all ingredients in the saucepan. Cover and simmer gently for 1-1½ hours or until the meat is tender.
Serves 6 [1576 kJ (375 Cal) per serve].

Microwave
Reduce the water to 1 cup. Do not brown the meat. Place all ingredients in a microwave proof dish. Cover and cook on 70% power for 15 minutes, reduce to 50% power for 15 minutes.
Stand 5 minutes.

Photograph page 77

Curry Accompaniments

Quantities for 6 servings.

Bananas

2 bananas
3 Tbsp lemon juice
cinnamon

Peel the bananas and slice into rings. Pour over the lemon juice and sprinkle with cinnamon. Serve chilled.

Cucumber

10 cm cucumber
¼ cup natural low fat
  yoghurt
1 Tbsp finely chopped
  fresh mint

Peel the cucumber only if the skin is bitter, slice thinly. Mix the cucumber, yoghurt and mint. Serve chilled.

Rice

4 cups hot cooked rice
½ cup finely chopped
  celery
½ cup raisins

Mix the rice, celery and raisins together. Serve hot.

CELERY AND WALNUT STUFFED LAMB

Roasting meat on a rack allows any fat to drain away — yet the lamb remains tender and full of flavour.

1 lean leg of lamb, boned
1 cup water
2 Tbsp water

2 Tbsp flour
freshly ground black pepper

Stuffing:

½ cup finely chopped celery, including leaves
1 onion, finely chopped
1 Tbsp finely chopped fresh herbs or ½ tsp dried mixed herbs

¼ cup finely chopped walnuts
¾ cup fresh wholemeal breadcrumbs
freshly ground black pepper
3-5 Tbsp water

Remove all visible fat from the meat. Place the stuffing on the meat, roll up and secure with string. Weigh the meat. Place on a rack in a roasting pan. Bake at 220°C for 20 minutes to seal the juices. Reduce the heat to 190°C and cook a further 20 minutes per 500g. Remove the meat from the roasting pan and keep warm. Drain all the fat from the pan. Add the first measure of water and heat the pan gently, stir to remove all cooked-on meat juices. Blend the second measure of water and flour to a paste, gradually add to the pan stirring continuously for 3-4 minutes or until thickened. Season to taste with pepper. Slice the meat and serve hot with the gravy.
Allow 125 g per serving.
[1017 kJ (242 Cal) per serve].

Stuffing:

Mix the celery, onion, herbs, walnuts, breadcrumbs and pepper together. Add enough water until the mixture holds together.

Photograph: Lamb Curry with Accompaniments (p.74).

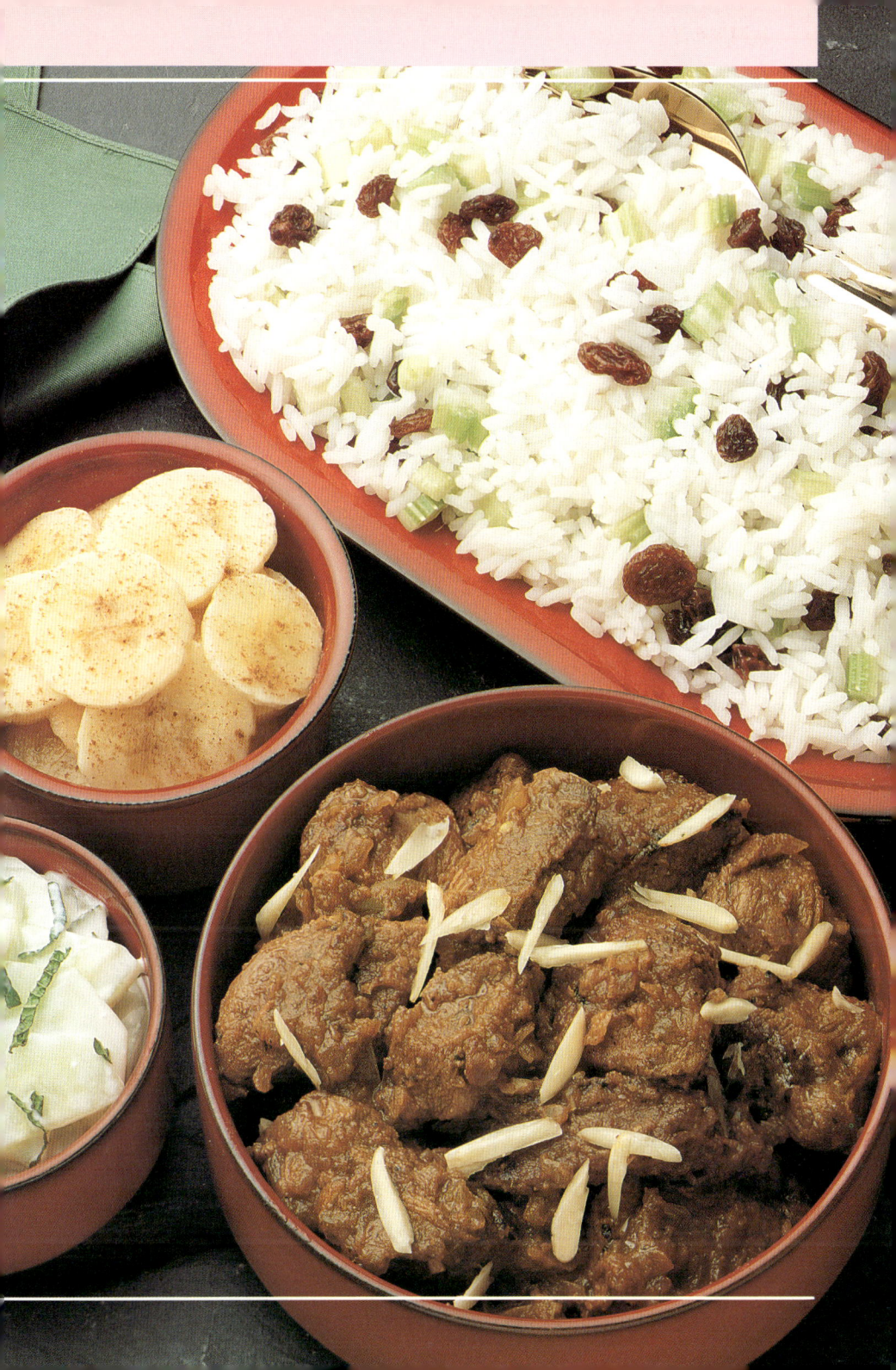

VEAL FLORENTINE

Although parmesan cheese is not low in fat, only a small amount is required to achieve a desirable cheesey taste. By selecting a lean meat cut and using non-fat milk this recipe is still low in fat without sacrificing flavour.

1 bunch (300 g)
   spinach or silverbeet
freshly ground black
   pepper
¼ tsp ground nutmeg
500 g lean veal
   schnitzel

6 tomatoes, sliced
   thickly
1 Tbsp grated
   parmesan cheese
¼ cup fresh wholemeal
   breadcrumbs

Cheese Sauce

1 Tbsp polyunsaturated
   oil
1 Tbsp flour
1 cup non-fat milk

¼ cup grated
   parmesan cheese
freshly ground black
   pepper

Wash the spinach and remove the stalks. Chop finely. Cook the spinach in a saucepan for 5 minutes, stirring regularly. Drain well, pressing out all the water. Season with pepper and nutmeg. Flatten the schnitzels with a rolling pin. Remove all visible fat and cut into strips. Heat in a non-stick frying pan and saute the meat until lightly browned. Place the tomatoes in an 8 cup-capacity casserole dish. Top with the spinach and then the meat. Pour the cheese sauce over and sprinkle with the parmesan cheese and breadcrumbs. Bake at 200°C for 10-15 minutes or until warmed through and golden brown.

Cheese Sauce

Heat the oil in a small saucepan. Add the flour and mix well. Gradually add the milk and parmesan cheese, stir continuously until thickened. Season generously with pepper.
Serves 6 [1145 kJ (273 Cal) per serve].

Microwave

Cover and cook the spinach on 100% power for 3½-4 minutes. Cook the meat on 70% power for 5-7 minutes. Stir once during cooking. Cook the assembled Florentine on 100% power for 4-5 minutes. Stand 5 minutes. Grill to brown the top if wished.

To make the cheese sauce blend the oil, flour, parmesan cheese and pepper together. Gradually add the milk, stirring until smooth. Cook on 100% power for 3-4 minutes, stirring once during cooking.

FRUITY PORK STIR-FRY

Take care not to overcook pork, and retain as many natural juices as possible. The fruits and vegetables add fibre, minerals and vitamins for a well-balanced meal in itself.

500 g lean pork schnitzel
¼ cup sherry
1 Tbsp honey
1 large red skinned apple, cored and cut into wedges
1 cup sliced celery
½ cup whole kernel corn
¼ cup sultanas
freshly ground black pepper
3 cups finely shredded cabbage
1 tsp cornflour

Remove all visible fat from the meat and cut into 2cm wide strips. Combine the meat with the sherry and honey. Marinate for 1 hour. Drain the meat, reserving the marinade and saute 3-4 minutes in a non-stick frying pan or lightly oiled wok. Add the apple, celery, corn, sultanas and pepper. Stir-fry 4-6 minutes or until vegetables are tender but still slightly crisp. Add the cabbage and stir-fry 1-2 minutes. Mix the cornflour and reserved marinade to a paste. Add to the frying pan, stir and heat 2-3 minutes or until thickened. Serve immediately. Serves 4 [1 429 kJ (340 Cal) per serve].

PORK AND PRUNES

2/9/89 - Philippa   easy to
         Robin   prepare -
         Gwyn   very fast

The wine and prunes add flavour and richness to this dish without adding fat or calories. High in fibre and minerals, prunes are a valuable addition.

2 lean pork fillets (500 g)
1 onion, finely chopped
1 cup red wine
1 Tbsp finely chopped
   fresh marjoram or 1
   tsp dried marjoram
1 cup water

¾ cup pitted prunes
¼ cup natural low fat
   yoghurt
2 Tbsp red currant jelly
freshly ground black
   pepper

Remove all visible fat from the pork and cut into 3cm wide slices. Brown in a non-stick frying pan. (It is easier to brown a few pieces at a time than all at once.) Add the onion, wine, marjoram and water. Cover and simmer gently for 15-20 minutes. Add the prunes and simmer another 10 minutes. Stir in the yoghurt, red currant jelly and season generously with pepper.
Serves 4 [1519 kJ (362 Cal) per serve].

Microwave

Reduce the water to ½ cup. Do not brown the meat. Place the pork, onion, wine, marjoram and water in a microwave proof casserole dish. Cover and cook on 70% power for 10-12 minutes. Add the prunes and cook on 70% power for 2-3 minutes. Mix 1 Tbsp cornflour and 1 Tbsp of water to a paste. Add the cornflour paste, yoghurt, red currant jelly and pepper to the casserole. Mix well. Cook on 70% power for 2-3 minutes or until the sauce thickens. Stand 5 minutes.

LAMB NOISETTES WITH APPLE AND MINT PUREE

The refreshing tang of mint and apple is an ideal lamb accompaniment. If time is limited, use middle loin chops. Remove the visible fat, leave the bone in.

2 cups peeled, cored and chopped apples
½ cup water
6 lean loin chops

½ cup fresh mint leaves
freshly ground black pepper
2 Tbsp natural low fat yoghurt

Place the apples and water in a saucepan. Cover and simmer for 15 minutes or until softened. Remove all visible fat from the meat, cut the thin layer of meat from the bone, leaving it attached to the eye of the chop. Remove the bone and wrap the thin meat layer around the eye of the chop. Secure with a toothpick. Puree the undrained apple, mint, pepper and yoghurt. Thin with water to preferred consistency. Fry the meat in a non-stick frying pan for 3 minutes each side or until they are cooked to your preference. Serve noisettes with the hot sauce.
Serve 4 [1351 kJ (322 Cal) per serve].

Microwave
Reduce the water to ¼ cup. Cover and cook the apples and water on 100% power for 5-6 minutes.

GOLDEN PORK

*2/8/89 Gwyn good - a
a self successful
combination*

An unusual but successful combination of fruit and vegetables suitable for a family dinner. Satisfying and so delicious.

4 lean pork butterfly
  steaks (500 g)
1 cup unsweetened
  apple juice
½ cup water
2 Tbsp soy sauce
½ tsp ground ginger

2 medium kumara,
  peeled and sliced
2 apples, peeled, cored
  and sliced
1 Tbsp flour
1 Tbsp water

Remove all visible fat from the meat and cut each steak in half. Brown the meat in a non-stick frying pan. (It is easier to brown a few pieces at a time than all at once). Place the browned meat in a large casserole dish. Add the apple juice, water, soy sauce, ginger and kumara. Cover and bake at 160°C for 1 hour, add the apples and cook a further ½ hour. Drain the juice from the casserole into a small saucepan. Mix the flour and water to a paste. Add to the juice and heat gently until thickened. Arrange pork, apple and kumara on a serving plate. Pour the sauce over.
Serves 4 [1319 kJ (314 Cal) per serve].

Microwave
Brown the meat and prepare casserole as instructed. Cover and cook on 70% power for 15 minutes. Add the apples and cook on 70% power for 8-10 minutes or until the kumara and apples are tender. Thicken the drained juices on 100% power for 2-3 minutes.

Photograph opposite page

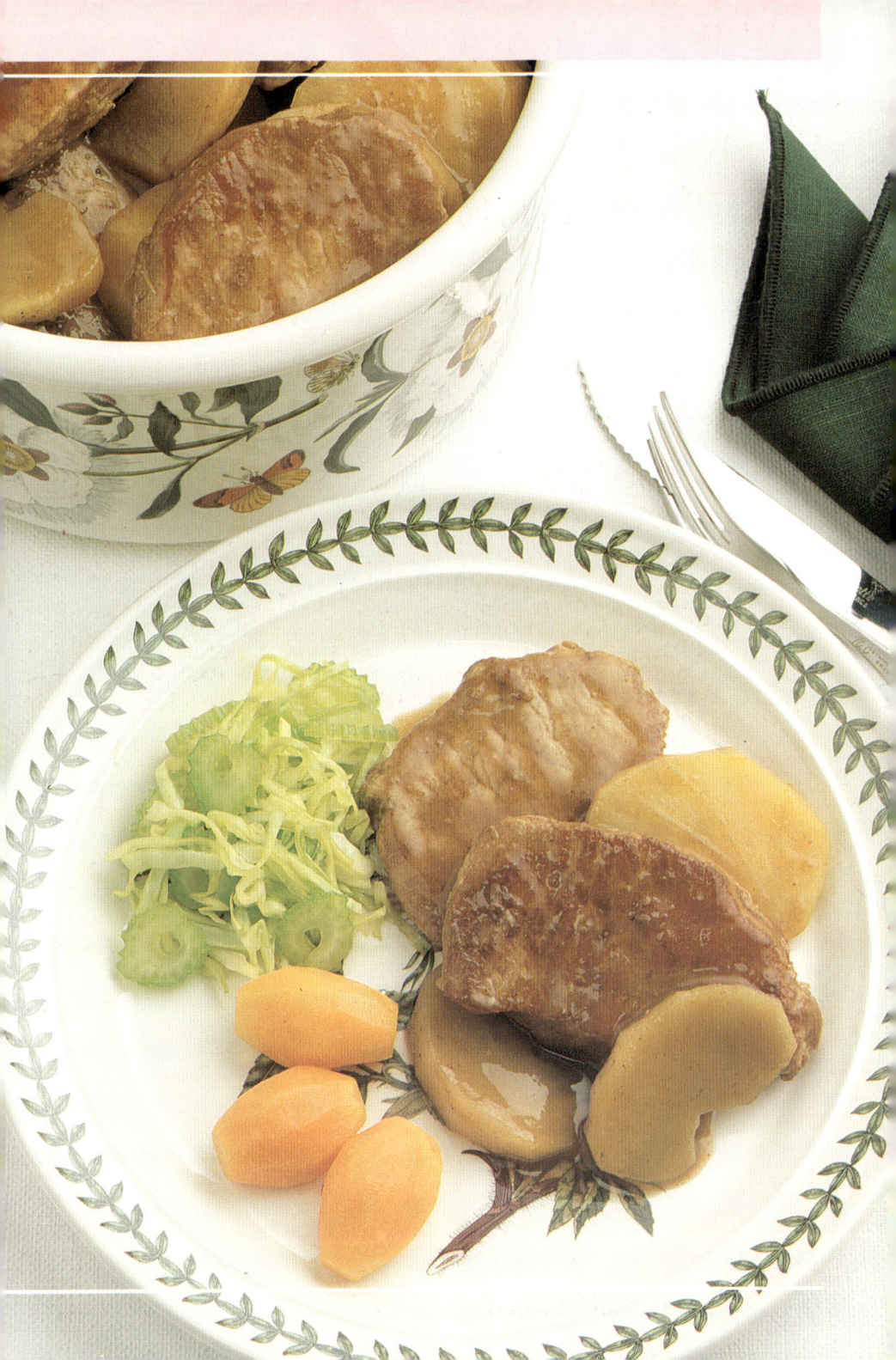

COTTAGE PIE

This family favourite helps meat go a little further.
To keep salt intake down use tinned products with
"no added salt" when available.

500 g cooked lean
   lamb
400 g tin whole peeled
   tomatoes
1 Tbsp Worcestershire
   sauce
1 Tbsp tomato paste

1 tsp dried basil or
   1 Tbsp chopped
   fresh basil
1 onion, roughly
   chopped
freshly ground black
   pepper
3 cups cooked mashed
   potato

In a food processor fitted with a metal blade, finely
chop the meat and set aside. Place the undrained
tomatoes, Worcestershire sauce, tomato paste,
basil, onion and pepper in the food processor and
blend until smooth. Combine with the chopped
meat and turn into 20cm square pie dish. Cover
with the mashed potato. Bake at 180°C for 30-35
minutes or until golden brown.
Serves 6 [1236 kJ (294 Cal) per serve].

Microwave
Assemble as instructed and sprinkle with paprika.
Cook, uncovered, on 100% power for 10-12
minutes. Stand 4 minutes.

CITRUS PORK ROLLS

Almost any fruit will combine successfully with pork but the refreshing tang of oranges enhances the flavour of this meat during cooking — as well as adding plenty of vitamin C

1 cup fresh wholemeal breadcrumbs
1 onion, finely chopped
¼ cup raisins
1 tsp grated orange rind
1 tsp fresh thyme or ½ tsp dried thyme
¼ cup freshly squeezed orange juice
4 lean pork schnitzels (500 g)

½ cup freshly squeezed orange juice
½ cup water
freshly ground black pepper
1 tsp cornflour
1 Tbsp water

Garnish:
orange slices
fresh thyme

Mix the breadcrumbs, onion, raisins, orange rind, thyme and first measure of orange juice together. Remove all visible fat from the meat and spread with the filling. Roll up and secure with toothpicks or string. Heat a non-stick frying pan and brown the rolls. Add the second measure of orange juice, first measure of water and pepper. Cover and simmer 20-25 minutes. Remove the rolls and discard the toothpicks or string. Keep warm. Mix the cornflour and second measure of water to a paste. Add to the pan and stir until thickened. Pour over the rolls and serve garnished with orange and thyme. Serves 4 [1449 kJ (345 Cal) per serve].

PINEAPPLE MEATBALLS

A family favourite with a difference. The wheatgerm adds fibre and vitamins as well as a crunchy texture. The spicy fruit sauce adds extra tang. Be sure the mince is lean to keep the fat content low.

220 g tin unsweetened
   crushed pineapple
400 g lean minced beef
1 onion, finely chopped
1½-2 Tbsp chilli sauce
freshly ground black
   pepper
1 egg

½ cup wheatgerm
wheatgerm to coat
1½ cups water
1 Tbsp soy sauce
1½-2 Tbsp chilli sauce
1 Tbsp cornflour
freshly ground black
   pepper

Drain the pineapple, reserve the juice. Mix the drained pineapple, mince, onion, first measure of chilli sauce, pepper, egg and wheatgerm together. Shape into small balls, flatten and coat with wheatgerm. Place in a single layer in a roasting dish and bake at 180°C for 20-25 minutes or until golden brown. Turn during cooking. Remove the meatballs and keep warm. Drain all the fat from the roasting pan. Add the water, soy sauce and second measure of chilli sauce to the roasting pan. Heat, stirring to remove any cooked-on meat juices. Mix the cornflour and pineapple juice to a paste. Add to the roasting pan and heat until thickened. Season to taste with pepper. Pour over the meatballs.
Serves 5 [901 kJ (215 Cal) per serve].

SWISS STEAK

*A popular casserole-type dish which is best
prepared the day before and left to marinate
overnight.*

500 g lean blade steak   ½ tsp dry mustard
1 Tbsp flour   2 Tbsp tomato sauce
½ tsp ground ginger   2 Tbsp vinegar
½ tsp curry powder   2 Tbsp sherry
½ tsp mixed spice   ½ cup water

Remove all visible fat from the meat and cut into
bite-sized pieces. Place all the ingredients in a
casserole dish. Mix well and marinate in the
refrigerator for 3-4 hours or overnight.
Cover and bake at 160°C for 2-2½ hours
or until the meat is tender.
Serves 4 [934 kJ (223 Cal) per serve].

Microwave
Cover and cook on 70% power for 15 minutes,
reduce to 50% power for 30 minutes.
Stand 5 minutes.

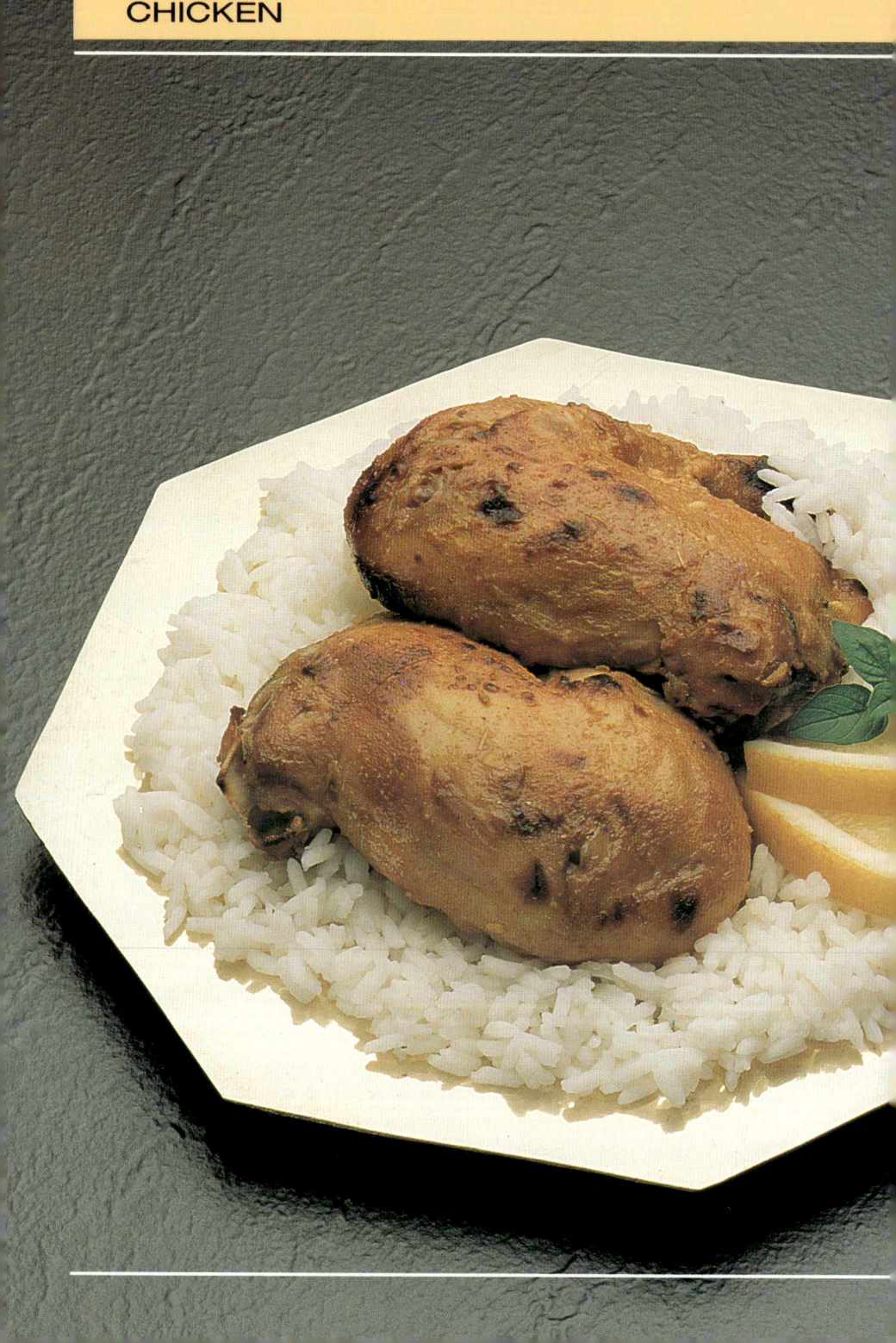

CHICKEN

Chicken is a good source of high quality protein which is naturally low in fat. Any fat which lies under the skin can easily be removed before cooking. Being readily available, popular with all ages and suitable for all occasions chicken, is a family favourite. In the recipes that follow the delicate flavour of chicken lends itself well to the use of fruit, with fresh herbs and spices used occasionally to enhance the mild taste.

Photograph: Tandoori Chicken (p.90).

TANDOORI CHICKEN

The yoghurt and spices in this recipe help tenderise the chicken and give a spicy tang. Serve with brown rice and a green vegetable for a good balance of flavour and food value.

1.5 kg chicken pieces
2 cloves garlic, peeled
  and finely chopped
1 cup natural low fat
  yoghurt
1 tsp ground ginger

1 tsp paprika
1 tsp ground coriander
1 tsp cumin
¼ dry mustard
¼ tsp chilli powder

Remove the skin and all visible fat from the chicken. Mix the garlic, yoghurt, ginger, paprika, coriander, cumin, mustard, and chilli powder together. Cut a few slashes in the flesh of each chicken piece. Combine the chicken and yoghurt mixture and refrigerate overnight. Place on a wire rack in a roasting dish. Bake at 200° C for 30-35 minutes or until a dark golden brown. Baste frequently with the yoghurt mixture during baking. Alternatively barbeque, turning and basting frequently. Serve hot or cold.
Serves 6 [717 kJ (171 Cal) per serve].

Photograph page 88.

LEEK AND PRUNE CHICKEN

*The prunes and leeks in this dish not only
complement the chicken in flavour and texture, but
add food value in the form of fibre and important
vitamins and minerals.*

4 boneless chicken
  breasts (500 g)
2 cups finely chopped
  leeks
¾ cup roughly
  chopped prunes

¼ tsp grated nutmeg
freshly ground black
  pepper
1 cup white wine
¼ cup natural low fat
  yoghurt

Remove the skin and all visible fat from the chicken.
Spread half the leeks over the base of a casserole
dish. Mix the remaining leeks, prunes, nutmeg and
pepper together. Fill each chicken breast with one
quarter of the prune mixture. Place the filled
chicken breasts on top of the leeks. Add the wine.
Cover and bake at 180°C for 25-30 minutes or until
the chicken and leeks are tender. Stir in the
yoghurt. Season with pepper.
Serves 4 [1205 kJ (287 Cal) per serve].

Microwave
Cover and cook on 70% power for 8-10 minutes.
Stir in the yoghurt and cook on 70% power for one
minute. Stand 4 minutes.

CHICKEN AND CELERY LOAF

This loaf is low in fat yet tasty and filling. The beans add flavour and texture as well as fibre and B vitamins. Serve it with a salad and vegetables of contrasting crunchy texture.

¾ cup uncooked
  kidney beans
3 stalks celery,
  including leaves,
  roughly chopped
2 eggs
2 Tbsp non-fat milk

freshly ground black
  pepper
1 cup fresh wholemeal
  breadcrumbs
2 cups roughly
  chopped raw
  chicken meat

Soak the beans in water overnight. Drain. Bring them to the boil in fresh water and simmer 45-50 minutes or until the beans are soft. Drain. Place the celery, eggs, milk and pepper in a food processor fitted with a metal blade. Process until well mixed. Combine the celery mixture, kidney beans, breadcrumbs and chicken together, adding extra milk to bind if necessary. Turn into a lightly greased 17 x 10cm loaf tin. Bake at 190°C for 35-40 minutes or until set and golden brown. Slice thinly and serve hot or cold.
Serves 6 [1089 kJ (259 Cal) per serve].

Note: A 310 g tin of kidney beans may be substituted for the soaked and cooked beans. Drain and rinse thoroughly.

Microwave
Place the soaked beans in boiling water and cook on 100% power for 20 minutes. Stand 10 minutes. Drain. Prepare the loaf as instructed. Turn into a lightly greased 19cm diameter microwave proof ring mould. Elevate and cook on 70% power for 14-16 minutes or until the mixture is set and leaves the side of the mould. Stand for 10 minutes before turning out.

CHILLI CHICKEN

This recipe helps a little chicken meat go a long way by combining it with other protein foods like rice, nuts and eggs. The vegetables, nuts and rice also add fibre and important vitamins and minerals, to make a complete well-balanced meal in itself.

1 cup brown rice
1 Tbsp polyunsaturated oil
1 onion, roughly chopped
1 clove garlic, peeled and finely chopped
2 cups roughly chopped cooked and skinned chicken
½ cup frozen peas

¼ cup roughly chopped almonds
¼ cup finely chopped fresh parsley
¼ tsp chilli powder
¼ cup water
2 tomatoes, roughly chopped
2 hard boiled eggs, roughly chopped

Cook the brown rice in boiling water for 25-30 minutes, or until tender. Drain. Heat the oil in a large saucepan and saute the onion and garlic for 2-3 minutes or until the onion softens. Add the rice, chicken, peas, almonds, parsley, chilli powder and water. Cook for 5-10 minutes stirring continuously. Add the tomatoes and eggs and heat through. Serves 6 [1106 kJ (263 Cal) per serve].

Microwave

Place the rice and 3 cups boiling water in a large microwave proof bowl. Cook on 100% power for 20 minutes. Stand 10 minutes. Drain. Omit the oil. In a large microwave proof bowl cover and cook the onion and garlic on 100% power for 2-3 minutes. Stir in the rice, chicken, peas, almonds, parsley, chilli powder and water. Cook on 100% power for 4 minutes. Add the tomatoes and eggs and cook on 100% power for 2 minutes.

PINEAPPLE AND CELERY CHICKEN

*Low fat yoghurt is used to thicken the sauce —
achieving a smooth creamy texture without adding
fat and too many calories.*

225 g tin unsweetened
   pineapple rings
1 cup fresh wholemeal
   breadcrumbs
½ cup finely chopped
   celery
1 egg
2 tsp finely chopped
   fresh sage or 1 tsp
   dried sage

4 boneless chicken
   breasts (500 g)
1 cup water
2 stalks celery, sliced
freshly ground black
   pepper
¼ cup natural low fat
   yoghurt

Drain the pineapple, reserving the juice. Finely
chop half the pineapple rings and mix with the
breadcrumbs, first measure of celery, egg and
sage. Remove the skin and all visible fat from the
chicken. Press one quarter of the filling mixture into
the pocket of each chicken breast. Place in a
roasting pan. Pour over reserved pineapple juice.
Bake at 180°C for 20-25 minutes or until golden
brown. Chop the remaining pineapple rings into
chunks. Add the pineapple and sliced celery to the
pan 5 minutes before the end of baking. Remove
the chicken, pineapple and celery from the pan
and keep warm. Add the water, stir over heat to
loosen the sediment. Reduce by boiling until the
sauce is thickened. Season with pepper and stir in
the yoghurt. Serve the chicken and sauce with the
pineapple and celery chunks.
Serves 4 [1193 kJ (284 Cal) per serve].

Microwave

Cover and cook on 70% power for 8-10 minutes or
until tender. Remove the chicken and keep warm.
Reduce the water to ⅓ cup. Mix 1 Tbsp cornflour
and 1 Tbsp of water to a paste. Add to the cooking
juices. Cook on 100% power for 1½-2 minutes.
Season with pepper and stir in the yoghurt. Cook
the celery and remaining chopped pineapple on
100% power for 2-3 minutes.

Photograph opposite page

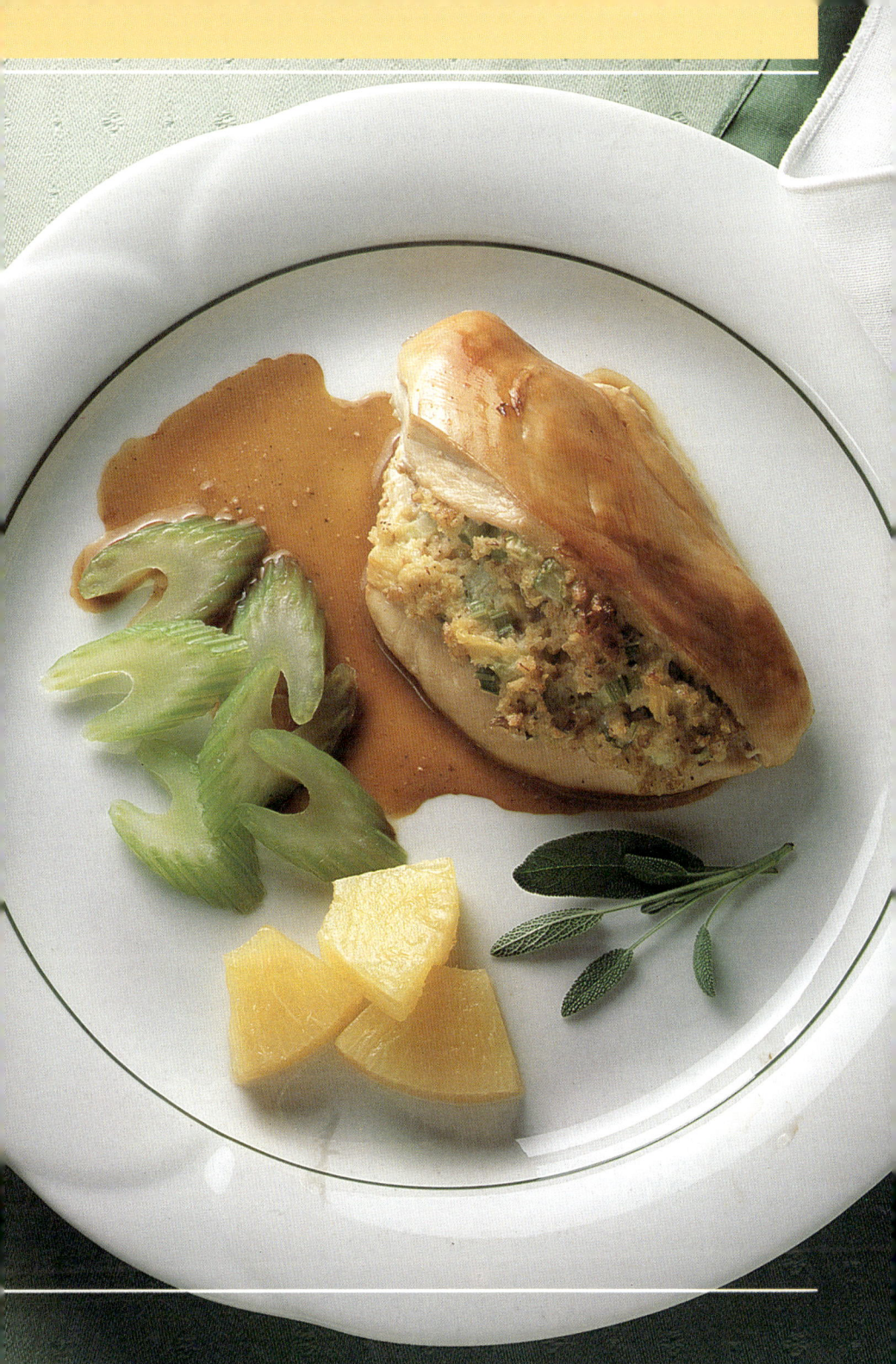

CHICKEN AND BEAN HOT POT

A substantial and satisfying family meal. The beans add fibre, B vitamins and minerals such as zinc and iron — yet are not high in fat or cholesterol.

¾ cup dried kidney
   beans
1 medium eggplant
1 tsp salt
1 kg chicken pieces
1 Tbsp polyunsaturated
   oil
1 onion, finely chopped
1 clove garlic, peeled
   and finely chopped

2 stalks celery,
   chopped
400 g tin whole peeled
   tomatoes
1 Tbsp finely chopped
   fresh basil or 1 tsp dried
   basil
freshly ground black
   pepper

Soak the beans in water overnight. Drain. Bring them to the boil in fresh water and simmer 45-50 minutes or until the beans are soft. Drain. Peel and dice the eggplant and sprinkle with salt. Stand for 30 minutes. Rinse thoroughly under cold running water. Drain. Remove the skin and visible fat from the chicken. Heat the oil in a frying pan and saute the onion, garlic, celery and eggplant for 3-4 minutes. Transfer to a large casserole dish. Saute the chicken for 5-6 minutes. Add the chicken, undrained tomatoes, beans, basil and pepper to the casserole dish. Bake covered at 180°C for 40-45 minutes or until the chicken is tender. Serves 6 [1065 kJ (254 Cal) per serve].

Note: A 310 g tin of kidney beans may be substituted for the soaked and cooked beans. Drain and rinse thoroughly.

Microwave

Place the soaked beans in boiling water and cook on 100% power for 20 minutes. Stand 10 minutes. Drain. Omit the oil. Prepare the eggplant and chicken as instructed. Cover and cook on 70% power for 15 minutes. Add the undrained tomatoes, beans, basil and pepper. Cover and cook on 70% power for 6-8 minutes or until the chicken is tender. Stand 4 minutes.

LEMON CHICKEN

A light tangy sauce which is quick and easy to prepare — combines well with the mild flavour of chicken.

1 kg chicken pieces
2 Tbsp lemon juice

Lemon Sauce

1 Tbsp polyunsaturated
  margarine
1 Tbsp flour
¾ cup chicken stock or
  white wine

1 Tbsp lemon juice
1 Tbsp brown sugar
1 Tbsp chopped chives
freshly ground black
  pepper

Remove the skin and all visible fat from the chicken. Sprinkle with the lemon juice and cover with foil. Bake at 180° C for 30-35 minutes or until the chicken is tender. Serve with lemon sauce.

Lemon Sauce

Melt the margarine in a small saucepan and stir in the flour. Gradually add the chicken stock, lemon juice and brown sugar. Heat gently stirring continuously for 3-4 minutes or until the sauce thickens. Stir in the chives. Season with pepper. Serves 4 [844 kJ (201 Cal) per serve].

Microwave

Cover and cook the chicken pieces on 70% power for 12-16 minutes. Stand 4 minutes.

Lemon Sauce

Melt the margarine on 100% power for 20 seconds. Stir in the flour. Gradually add the chicken stock, lemon juice and brown sugar, stirring until smooth. Cook on 100% power for 3-4 minutes or until the sauce thickens. Stir once during cooking. Stir in the chives. Season with pepper.

CHICKEN AND BROCCOLI CASSEROLE

A smooth creamy sauce can be achieved without butter and cream. Use instead a little polyunsaturated oil and non-fat milk — low in fat yet just as tasty.

1.2 kg whole chicken
1 onion, roughly
   chopped
1 carrot, roughly
   chopped
3 bay leaves
2 cups broccoli florets
1 cup sliced
   mushrooms

1 Tbsp polyunsaturated
   oil
2 Tbsp flour
⅓ cup non-fat milk
   powder
⅓ cup sherry
1 Tbsp finely chopped
   fresh marjoram or
   1 ½ tsp dried
   marjoram
freshly ground black
   pepper

Remove the giblets and any excess fat from the chicken. Place the chicken, onion, carrot and bay leaves in a large saucepan. Cover with water and simmer for 45-50 minutes or until juices run clear when inserted with a skewer. Reserve 1 ½ cups of the cooking liquid. Discard the skin and bone and roughly chop the chicken. Place the chicken, broccoli and mushrooms in a large casserole dish. Blend the oil, flour and milk powder together. Gradually add the sherry and reserved cooking liquid, blending until smooth. Add the marjoram and season generously with pepper. Pour into the casserole dish. Bake at 180°C for 30-35 minutes. Serves 6 [857 kJ (204 Cal) per serve].

Microwave
Place the chicken, onion, carrot and bay leaves in a large microwave proof dish. Add 4 cups of boiling water. Cover and cook on 70% power for 25-30 minutes. Proceed as instructed. Cover and bake on 70% power for 7-8 minutes. Stir once during cooking. Stand 4 minutes.

APRICOT GINGER CHICKEN

A deliciously simple meal — the fruit and the subtle hint of ginger combine well with the delicate flavour of chicken. Low in fat yet high in flavour.

4 boneless chicken
  breasts (500 g)
425 g tin apricot nectar
3 cm piece root ginger,
  peeled and finely
  sliced

2 tsp cornflour
1 Tbsp water
2 spring onions,
  finely sliced

Remove the skin and visible fat from the chicken. Place the chicken, apricot nectar and ginger in a casserole dish. Cover and bake at 180° C for 20-25 minutes or until tender. Blend the cornflour and water to a paste and add to the casserole. Return to the oven for 5 minutes or until the sauce thickens. Sprinkle with the spring onions.
Serves 4 [893 kJ (213 Cal) per serve].

Note: For an economical chicken dish use chicken pieces.

Microwave
Cover and cook on 70% power for 8-10 minutes or until tender. Blend the cornflour and water to a paste. Add to the casserole and cook on 100% power for 1-2 minutes or until the sauce thickens. Stand 4 minutes. Sprinkle with the spring onions.

CHICKEN AND VEGETABLE TOSS

A meal ready in minutes, a stir-fry is easy to prepare. Quick cooking methods retain the colour, texture and food value of the vegetables.

4 chicken pieces
   eg. thighs (1 kg)
1 Tbsp polyunsaturated
   oil
1 cup sliced green
   beans
1 cup sliced carrots
¼ cup water

1 cup bean sprouts
1 cup sliced
   mushrooms
2 Tbsp finely chopped
   fresh parsley
¼-½ tsp Chinese five
   spice
freshly ground black
   pepper

Remove the skin, visible fat and bone from the chicken. Cut into bite-sized pieces. Heat the oil in a large frying pan or wok. Stir-fry the chicken for 5-10 minutes or until white and cooked through. Add the beans, carrots and water. Cook stirring for 5-10 minutes or until tender but still slightly crunchy. Add the bean sprouts, mushrooms, parsley, Chinese five spice and pepper. Cook a further 3-4 minutes or until warmed through.
Serves 4 [944 kJ (225 Cal) per serve].

Photograph opposite page

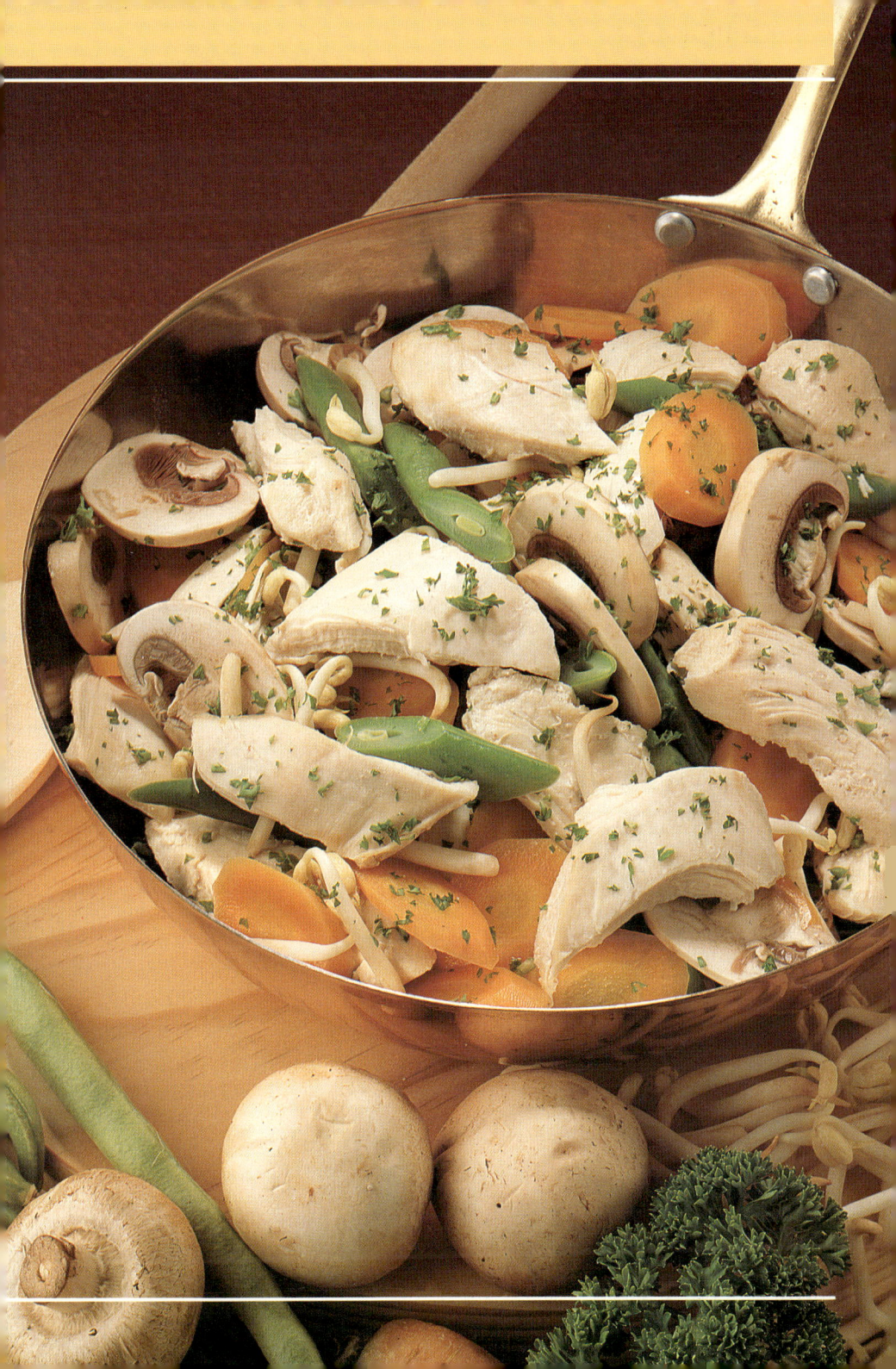

SESAME CHICKEN

Marinades have a wonderful effect on tenderness, moisture and flavour. Without adding oil this marinade retains the low fat content of chicken.

1 kg chicken pieces
1 Tbsp soy sauce
1 Tbsp honey
1 Tbsp tomato paste
½ cup red wine

1 Tbsp sesame seeds
1 clove garlic, peeled
    and finely chopped
1 tsp ground ginger
    freshly ground black
        pepper

Remove the skin and all visible fat from the chicken. Make the marinade by combining the remaining ingredients. Place the marinade and chicken in a shallow oven proof dish and marinate 2-3 hours or overnight. Bake at 180°C for 30-40 minutes or until tender. Baste frequently during cooking. Alternatively, barbeque turning and basting frequently.
Serves 4 [871 kJ (207 Cal) per serve].

Microwave
Cover and cook on 70% power for 12-15 minutes or until tender. Turn once during cooking. Stand 4 minutes.

Photograph page 171.

CHICKEN STRUDEL

Filo pastry is light in texture and not difficult to use. Be sure to handle it quickly so it does not dry out. Use fresh asparagus when in season for added vitamins and minerals.

¼ cup natural low fat yoghurt
340 g tin asparagus bits, drained
2 cups roughly chopped, cooked and skinned chicken
1 Tbsp finely chopped fresh thyme or 1½ tsp dried thyme

2 Tbsp sherry
freshly ground black pepper
4 sheets filo pastry
2 Tbsp polyunsaturated oil

Mix the yoghurt, asparagus, chicken, thyme, sherry and pepper together. Place one sheet of the filo pastry on a clean flat surface. Brush sparingly with oil. Place the second sheet of pastry on top of this. Brush with oil. Continue layering until you have used the 4 sheets. Place the filling along the length of pastry. Roll up, folding the end in, to form a long tube. Make light diagonal slashes on the surface. Bake at 200°C for 15-20 minutes or until golden brown.
Serves 5 [1011 kJ (241 Cal) per serve].

Note: When asparagus is in season substitute the tin with 8-10 spears of fresh asparagus. Steam for 6-8 minutes or until tender. Roughly chop.

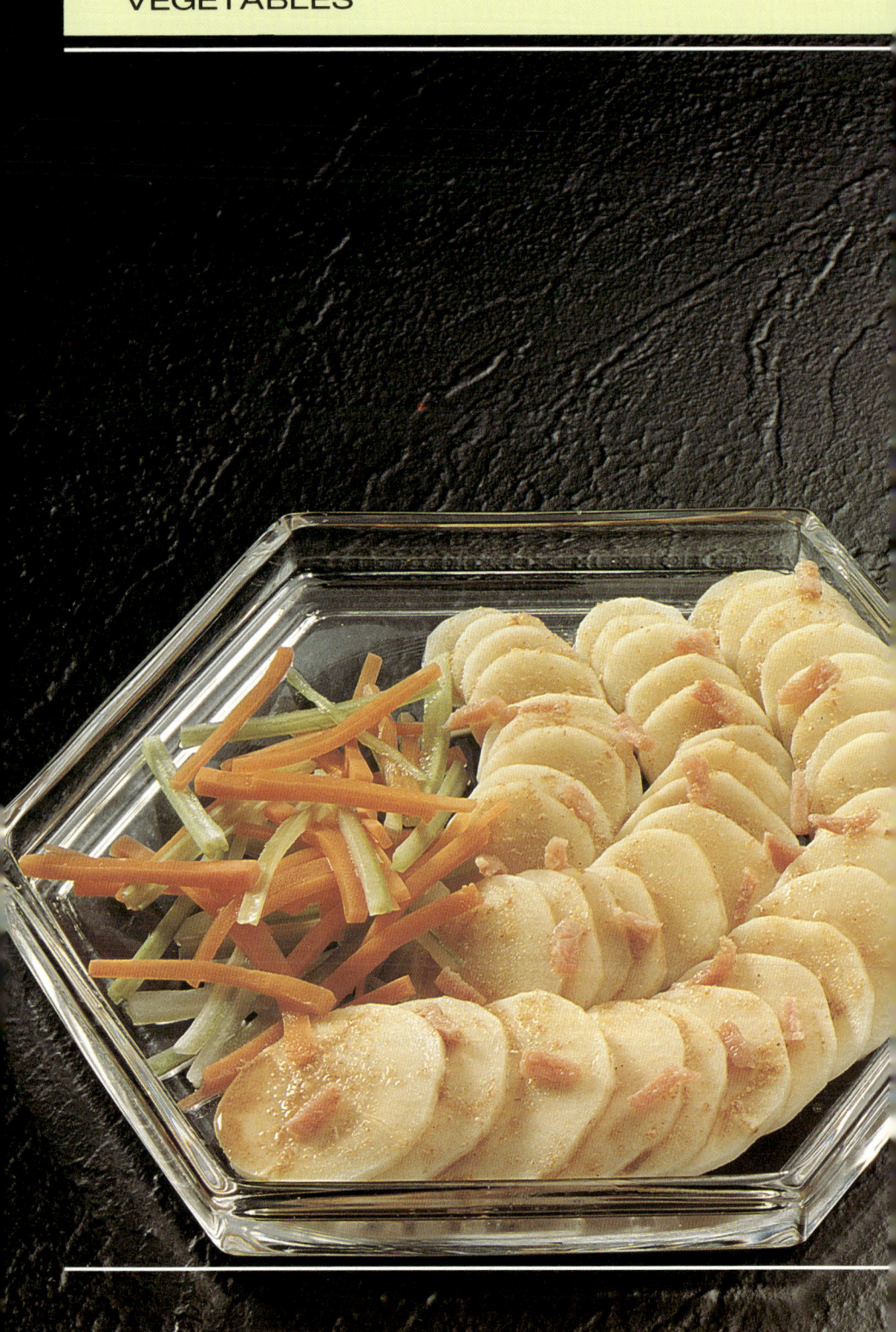

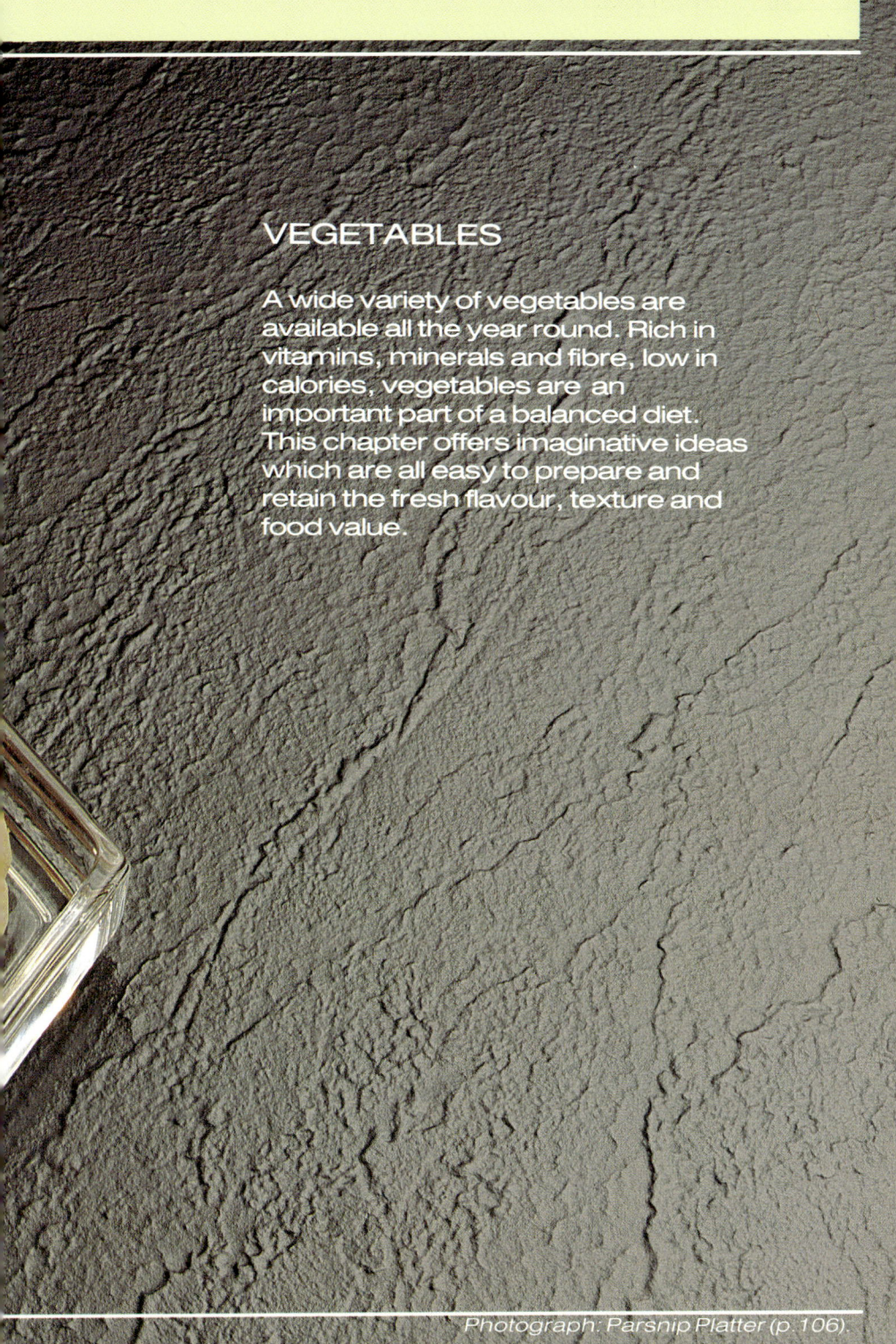

VEGETABLES

A wide variety of vegetables are available all the year round. Rich in vitamins, minerals and fibre, low in calories, vegetables are an important part of a balanced diet. This chapter offers imaginative ideas which are all easy to prepare and retain the fresh flavour, texture and food value.

Photograph: Parsnip Platter (p. 106).

PARSNIP PLATTER

Although parsnips taste sweet and starchy they are low in calories. Be sure to remove all fat from bacon. This will keep the fat content down without losing the flavour.

1 carrot
2 stalks celery
2 rashers lean bacon

2 medium parsnips,
 peeled and sliced
½ tsp ground cumin
1 Tbsp vinegar

Cut the carrots and celery into thin strips. Remove all visible fat and rind from the bacon, chop finely. Saute the bacon, parsnip and cumin in a non-stick frying pan for 6-8 minutes or until the parsnip is tender. Add the carrot and celery to the pan and stir-fry for 3-4 minutes or until the vegetables are tender but still slightly crisp. Add the vinegar and toss through. Serve immediately.
Serves 4 [360 kJ (86 Cal) per serve].

Microwave
Cover and cook the bacon, parsnip and cumin on 100% power for 5-6 minutes. Add the carrot and celery. Cook on 100% power for 2-3 minutes or until the vegetables are tender but still slightly crisp. Add the vinegar and toss through.

Photograph page 104

LEMON YAMS

The tangy flavour of lemon combines well with the mild sweet taste of yams. The small amount of brown sugar adds extra sweetness and crispness.

500 g yams
3 Tbsp lemon juice

1 tsp grated lemon rind
2 Tbsp brown sugar

Place the yams, lemon juice, lemon rind and
brown sugar in an ovenproof dish. Mix well.
Cover and bake at 180°C for 45-55 minutes or
until tender but still slightly crisp. Turn several
times during cooking.
Serves 6 [450 kJ (107 Cal) per serve].

Microwave
Cover and cook on 100% power for 12-14 minutes
or until tender but still slightly crisp. Turn several
times during cooking. Stand 3 minutes.

BEETROOT WITH HORSERADISH

*Beetroot is sweet, but not as high in calories as you
may think. Use low fat yoghurt and milk to keep the
fat content and calories down.*

4 medium beetroot
¼ cup natural low fat
  yoghurt
1 Tbsp horseradish
  sauce

3 Tbsp non-fat milk
freshly ground black
  pepper

Place the beetroot in a saucepan, cover with water
and bring to the boil. Simmer 30-40 minutes or until
tender. Drain. Remove the skins and discard. Cut
the beetroot into chunks. Keep warm. Mix the
yoghurt, horseradish, milk and pepper together.
Pour over the beetroot. Serve warm.
Serves 6 [104 kJ (25 Cal) per serve].

Microwave
Place the beetroot in a large microwave proof bowl.
Cover with boiling water and cook on 100% power
for 20 minutes or until tender. Prepare as instructed.
Cover and cook the beetroot and sauce on 100%
power for 1-2 minutes or until warmed through.

PUMPKIN PUREE

Purees of lightly cooked and seasoned vegetables complement any firm-textured main course. Pumpkin is slightly sweet, and high in vitamin A.

500 g pumpkin
¼ cup natural low fat
  yoghurt

freshly ground black
  pepper
¼ tsp freshly grated
  nutmeg

Peel and roughly chop the pumpkin. Steam or boil the pumpkin for 12-15 minutes or until tender. Puree with the yoghurt, pepper and nutmeg. Serve immediately.
Serves 4 [190 kJ (45 Cal) per serve].

Note: Use more yoghurt if the pumpkin is dry.

Microwave
Cover and cook on 100% power for 7-9 minutes, or until tender.

Photograph opposite page.

COURGETTES AND CHIVES

Courgettes, also known as zucchini, cook very quickly. Served immediately they will keep their colour and shape.

1 tsp polyunsaturated oil
6 small courgettes,
  sliced

½ tsp celery seeds
1 Tbsp chopped chives

Heat the oil in a frying pan. Add the courgettes and celery seeds. Toss together. Stir-fry 3-5 minutes. Sprinkle with chives before serving.
Serves 4 [94 kJ (22 Cal) per serve].

Microwave
Mix the oil, courgettes and celery seeds together in a microwave proof bowl. Cover and cook on 100% power for 3-4 minutes or until the courgettes are softened. Sprinkle with chives.

Photograph opposite page.

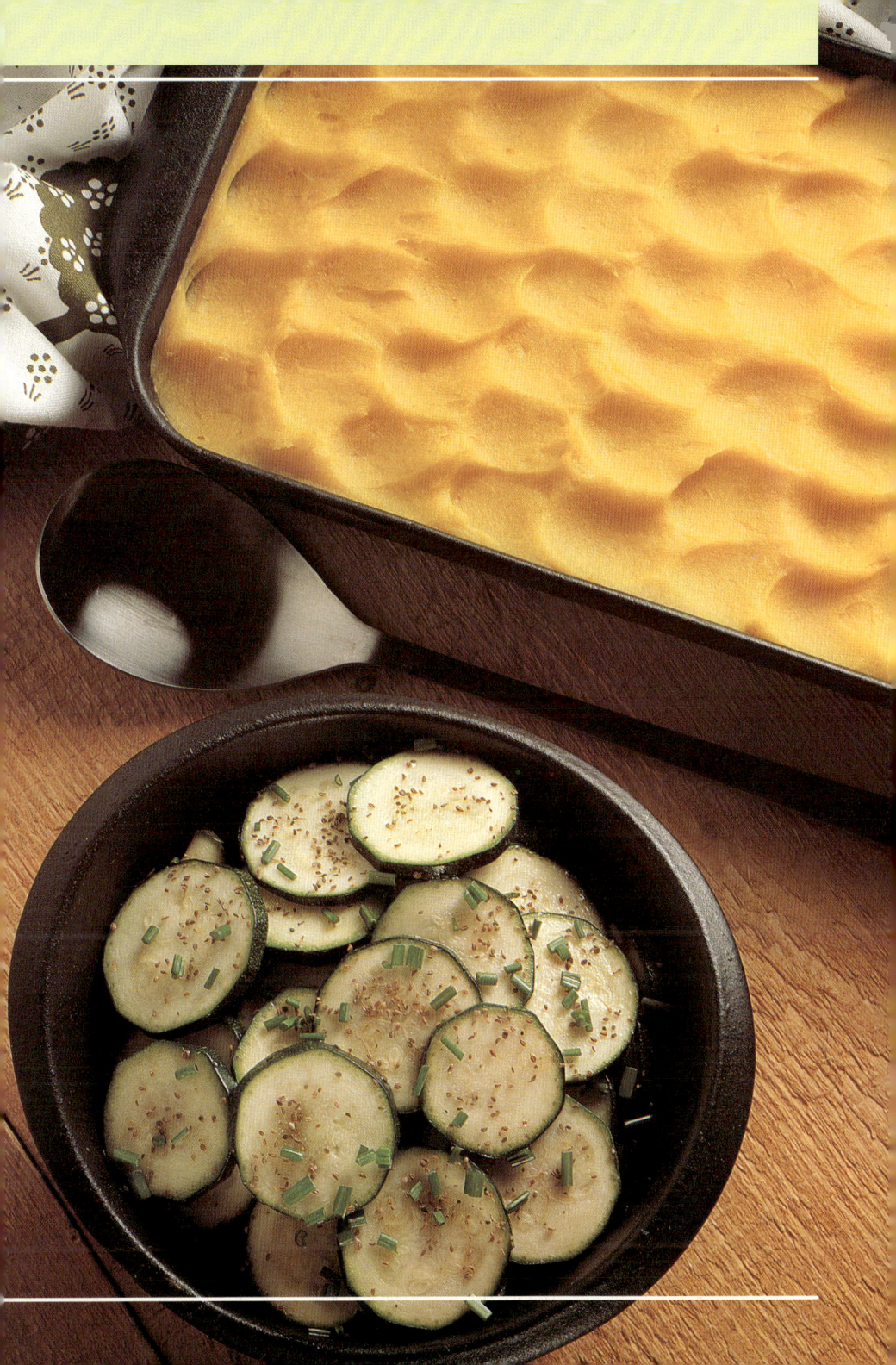

NUTTY BRUSSELS

Remember to treat all vegetables with care — keep cooking time to a minimum to retain their colour, texture and food value.

400 g Brussels sprouts
1 tsp polyunsaturated
  margarine

1 Tbsp flaked almonds
freshly ground black
  pepper

Trim off any damaged leaves. Cut a cross in the stem. Steam for 8-10 minutes or until tender. Place in a serving bowl, dot with margarine and sprinkle with almonds and pepper.
Serves 4 [262 kJ (62 Cal) per serve].

Microwave
Cover and cook on 100% power for 3-4 minutes or until tender.

CRISPY CABBAGE

Green vegetables are rich in fibre, vitamins and minerals, yet low in calories. Cook cabbage quickly using a little polyunsaturated oil, to keep its crunchy texture and food value.

1 tsp polyunsaturated
  oil
1 onion, finely chopped

¼ tsp Chinese five
  spice
4 cups finely shredded
  cabbage

Heat the oil in a large frying pan or wok. Saute the onion for 2-3 minutes or until softened. Add the Chinese five spice and cabbage. Cook 3-4 minutes, stirring continuously. Serve immediately.
Serves 4 [149 kJ (36 Cal) per serve].

Microwave
Place the oil, onion and Chinese five spice in a microwave proof dish. Cover and cook on 100% power for 2-3 minutes. Add the cabbage. Cover and cook on 100% power for 2 minutes.

MOUTHWATERING MUSHROOMS

Light and subtle in flavour. It is important not to overpower the delicate taste of mushrooms. Look out for low salt tomato paste when shopping.

2 Tbsp lemon juice
2 Tbsp finely chopped
   fresh parsley
1 Tbsp tomato paste
½ cup water

2 spring onions, finely
   chopped
¼ tsp ground coriander
250 g button
   mushrooms

Place all the ingredients in a saucepan. Mix well.
Bring to the boil and simmer 6-8 minutes.
Serve hot or cold.
Serves 4 [87 kJ (21 Cal) per serve].

Microwave
Reduce water to ¼ cup. Cover and cook on 100% power for 3-4 minutes.

CITRUS KUMARA

*Kumara is naturally sweet and fibre rich.
It combines well with citrus juices and spices.*

4 cups peeled and
   roughly chopped
   kumara
½ cup freshly
   squeezed orange
   juice

1 tsp grated orange rind
1 Tbsp honey
¼-½ tsp cinnamon
1 Tbsp sesame seeds

Place the kumara, orange juice, orange rind,
honey, cinnamon and sesame seeds in an
ovenproof dish. Mix well. Cover and bake at 180°C
for 30-40 minutes or until the kumara is tender.
Serves 6 [685 kJ (163 Cal) per serve].

Microwave
Cover and cook on 100% power for 9-12 minutes
or until the kumara is tender.

SUNFLOWER SEED BEANS

Sunflower seeds are similar to nuts in terms of food value — high in protein, vitamins and fibre. They also have a high polyunsaturated oil content. In this recipe they add extra flavour and crunchiness.

250 g green beans
2 large tomatoes,
  thickly sliced
1 Tbsp toasted
  sunflower seeds

1 tsp fresh thyme
freshly ground black
  pepper

Top and tail the beans and cut into 10cm lengths. Steam the beans for 5-8 minutes or until tender. Add the tomatoes and steam a further 2 minutes. Toss the beans, tomatoes, sunflower seeds, thyme and pepper together. Serve hot.
Serves 4 [168 kJ (40 Cal) per serve].

Microwave
Cover and cook the beans on 100% power for 3-4 minutes. Add the tomatoes, sunflower seeds, thyme and pepper. Cook on 100% power for 1-1½ minutes.

Photograph opposite page

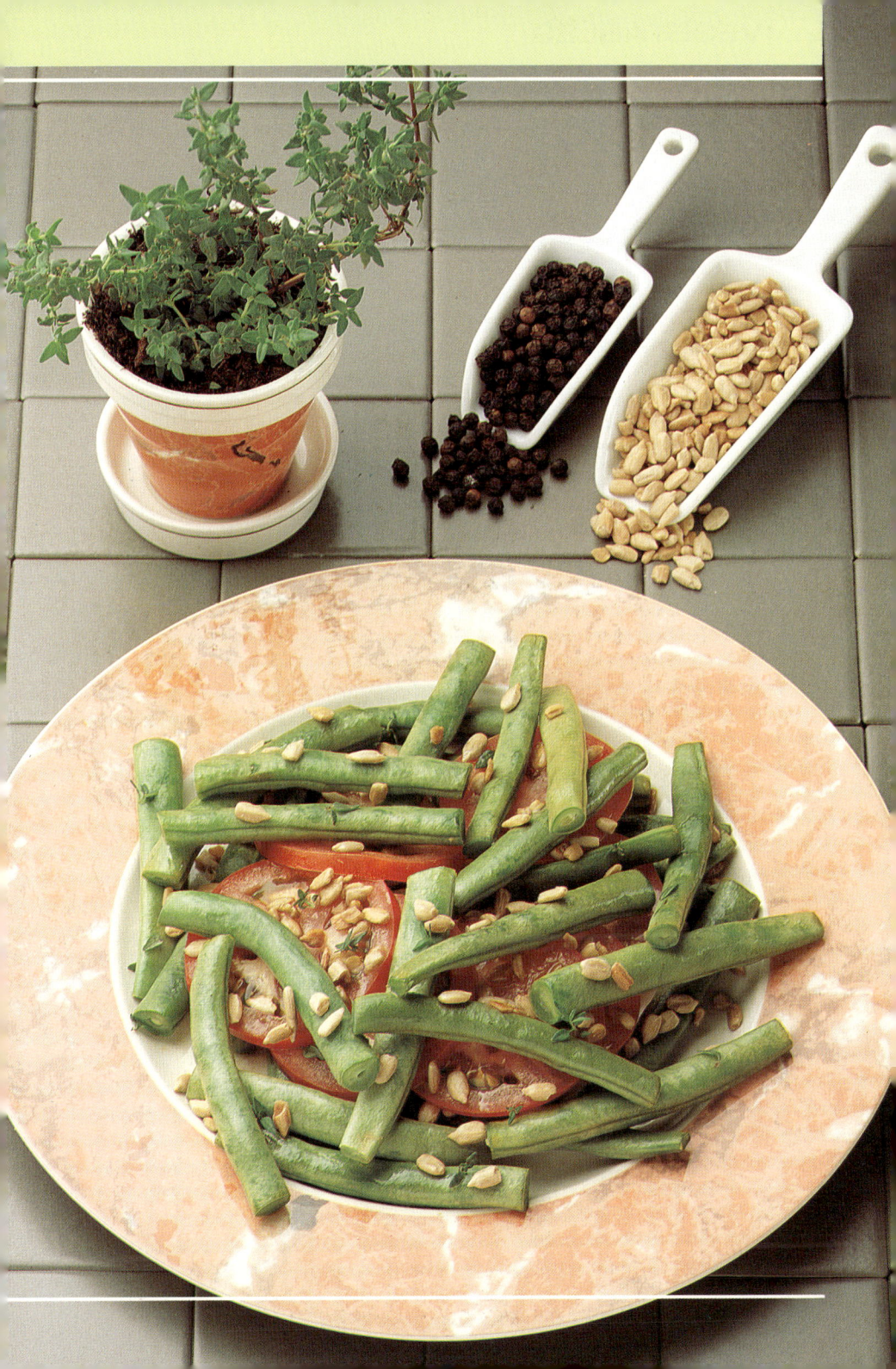

TANGY CARROTS

A popular vegetable for colour, versatility and flavour — suitable for every meal. High in fibre and a good source of vitamin A.

1½ cups water	1 Tbsp cornflour
4 medium carrots, sliced	1 Tbsp sugar
	1 Tbsp vinegar

Bring the water to the boil and add the carrots. Cover and simmer for 8-10 minutes or until tender. Drain, reserving 1 cup of the juice. In a saucepan mix the cornflour, sugar and vinegar to a paste. Gradually add the carrot juice, heating gently and stirring until thickened. Add the carrots and heat through. Serve hot.
Serves 4 [177 kJ (42 Cal) per serve].

Microwave
Reduce the water to 1 cup. Place the carrots and water in a microwave proof dish. Cover and cook on 100% power for 5-7 minutes or until tender. Drain, reserving the juice. Mix the cornflour, sugar and vinegar to a paste. Blend in the carrot juice and cook on 100% power for 2 minutes.
Add the carrots, cook on 100% power for 1 minute.

CRUNCHY CAULIFLOWER

This cauliflower dish is an economical and versatile accompaniment or a complete meal. The small amount of cheese adds flavour and texture and is a natural partner for this vegetable.

500 g (½ head) cauliflower
1 Tbsp polyunsaturated oil
1 onion, finely chopped
¼ cup fresh wholemeal breadcrumbs

2 Tbsp finely chopped fresh parsley
1-2 tsp caraway seeds
2 Tbsp grated parmesan cheese

Break the cauliflower into serving portions. Steam for 5-10 minutes or until tender but still slightly crisp. Place in an ovenproof dish and keep warm. Heat the oil in a frying pan, and saute the onion for 2-3 minutes. Add the breadcrumbs stir-frying until golden brown. Remove from the heat. Stir in the caraway seeds, parsley and parmesan cheese. Sprinkle over cauliflower. Grill for 3-5 minutes if wished.
Serves 4 (425 kJ (101 Cal) per serve].

Variation: Use broccoli in place of cauliflower, or a combination of both.

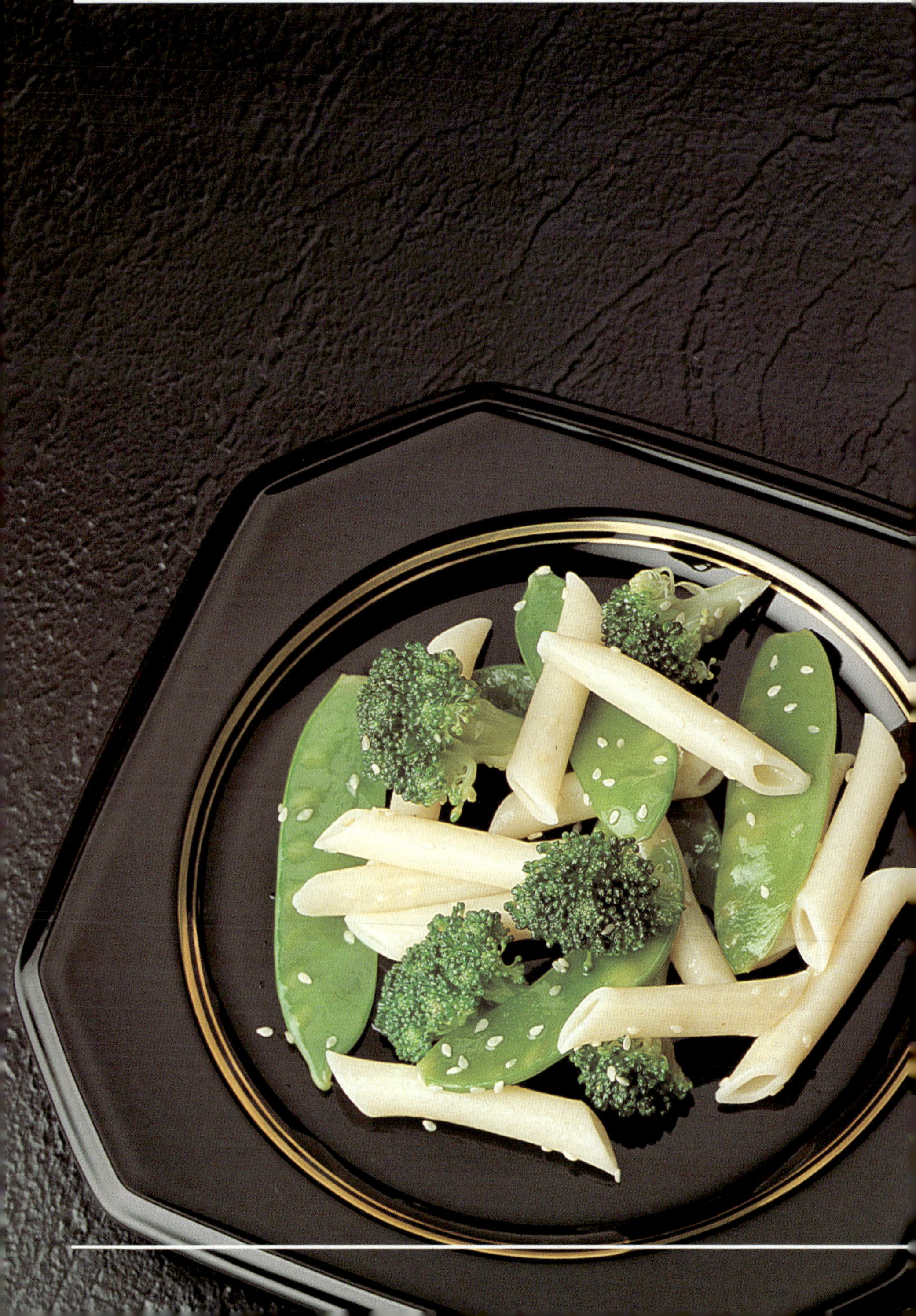

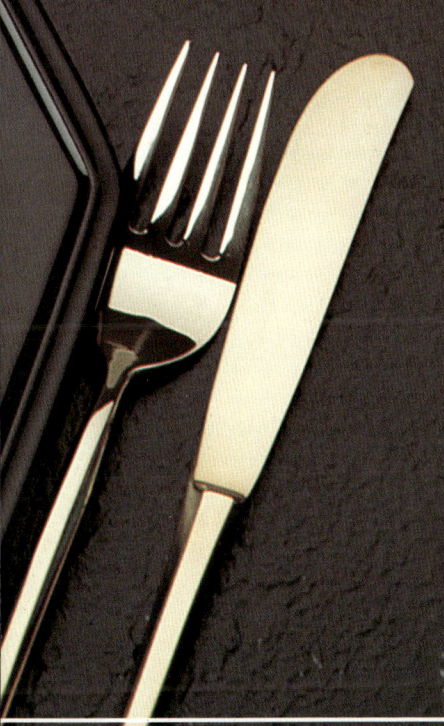

SALADS

For colour, variety, freshness and texture salads can be served regularly throughout the year. Salad can be an entree, an accompaniment to the main meal or a meal itself. This chapter offers some new salad combinations using crisp, fresh vegetables and fruit, packed with goodness and low in calories. A variety of light dressings, with fresh herbs and spices can be added for extra flavour.

Photograph: Pasta Salad with Sesame Dressing (p. 118).

PASTA SALAD WITH SESAME DRESSING

*Also known as mangetout, snow peas are
tender young peas that are eaten pod and all.
Take care not to overcook them so they keep
their bright green colour and crisp texture — an
ideal partner to pasta.*

1 cup snow peas
   (mangetout)
2 cups broccoli florets

1 ½ cups dried pasta
   (small tubes or
   macaroni elbows)

Sesame Dressing

1 Tbsp polyunsaturated
   oil
2 Tbsp lemon juice

2 tsp sesame seeds
freshly ground black
   pepper

Steam the snow peas and broccoli for 7-8 minutes
until tender but still slightly crisp. Cook the pasta
in a large saucepan of boiling water for 10-12
minutes or until tender. Drain well. Combine the
snow peas, broccoli, pasta and dressing.
Serve warm or chilled.

Sesame Dressing
In a screw top jar place the oil, lemon juice, sesame
seeds and pepper. Shake well.
Serves 4 [1178 kJ (281 Cal) per serve].

Microwave
Cover and cook the snow peas and broccoli on
100% power for 3½-4 minutes or until tender but
still slightly crisp. Bring a microwave proof bowl of
water to the boil, add the pasta and cook on 100%
power for 10-12 minutes or until tender. Drain well.

Photograph page 116

CURRIED POTATO SALAD

New potatoes can be very lightly cooked in their skins, then dressed and served while still warm. Without the usual high fat mayonnaise, this potato salad is not high in calories.

4 medium potatoes
3 spring onions, finely
   sliced

2 Tbsp sunflower seeds

Curry Dressing

¼ cup natural low fat
   yoghurt

¾ tsp curry powder
2 Tbsp non-fat milk

Scrub and boil the potatoes for 20-25 minutes or until tender. Drain and cut into bite-sized chunks. Combine with spring onions, sunflower seeds and dressing. Serve warm or chilled.

Curry Dressing
Mix the yoghurt, curry powder and milk together. Serves 4 [538 kJ (128 Cal) per serve].

Microwave
Scrub and pierce potatoes. Cook on 100% power for 10-12 minutes. Stand 5 minutes.

RED CABBAGE SLAW

Red cabbage is as high in vitamin C as the green varieties. It is best mixed with other ingredients as on its own it can have too strong a flavour.

225 g tin unsweetened crushed pineapple
½ cup raisins
2 cups finely shredded red cabbage

¼ cup chopped walnuts
2 Tbsp freshly squeezed orange juice
freshly ground black pepper

Drain the pineapple, reserving the juice. Place the raisins and pineapple juice in a small saucepan, simmer 5 minutes or until the raisins are plump. Cool. Combine the red cabbage, crushed pineapple, walnuts, orange juice, pepper, raisins and pineapple juice. Serve chilled.
Serves 4 [701 kJ (167 Cal) per serve].

Microwave
Cook the raisins and pineapple juice on 100% power for 2-3 minutes or until the raisins are plump.

TOMATO AND BASIL VINAIGRE

This dressing is low in calories, but still adds flavour and tang to a salad.

20 cm cucumber
4 tomatoes, finely sliced

1 red skinned onion, finely sliced

Basil Vinaigre

1 Tbsp finely chopped fresh basil
¼ cup spiced vinegar

½ tsp sugar
freshly ground black pepper

Peel the cucumber if the skin is bitter, slice finely.
Combine the cucumber, tomatoes and onion. Pour
the vinaigre over the salad. Refrigerate for 1-2 hours
before serving.

Basil Vinaigre
Stir the basil, vinegar, sugar and pepper together
until the sugar dissolves.
Serves 4 [167 kJ (40 Cal) per serve].

Photograph page 171

CARROT AND POPPYSEED SALAD

*Bean sprouts make a versatile, crunchy salad
ingredient. Sprouts are also high in vitamin C
and minerals.*

3 cups grated carrot   1 cup bean sprouts
1 cup sliced
    mushrooms

Poppyseed Dressing

1 tsp poppyseeds   1 tsp sugar
2 Tbsp lemon juice   freshly ground black
2 tsp polyunsaturated   pepper
    oil

Place the carrot, mushrooms and bean sprouts in a
bowl. Add the dressing and mix well.

Poppyseed Dressing
Mix the poppyseeds, lemon juice, oil, sugar and
pepper together.
Serves 4 [394 kJ (94 Cal) per serve].

SPINACH SALAD WITH LEMON MINT DRESSING

Spinach offers a change from the usual lettuce salad — and offers much in food value. High in vitamins, minerals and fibre. When teamed with foods high in vitamin C it is a rich source of iron.

1 bunch (300g) fresh
    spinach leaves

1 red skinned apple
1 cup alfalfa sprouts

Lemon Mint Dressing

2 medium lemons
4-5 sprigs of fresh mint
2 tsp sugar

2 Tbsp lemon juice
¼ cup spiced vinegar
freshly ground black
    pepper

Place spinach leaves on a serving platter. Cut the apple into wedges and mix into the spinach. Place alfalfa sprouts on the top. Pour the dressing over or serve separately.

Lemon Mint Dressing

Using a sharp knife, remove the rind from the lemon, taking as little pith as possible. Fit a food processor with a metal blade. With the motor running drop the lemon rind and mint down the feed tube. When the lemon and mint are very finely chopped add the sugar, lemon juice, vinegar and pepper. Continue processing until well mixed. Serves 4 [220 kJ (53 Cal) per serve].

Photograph opposite page

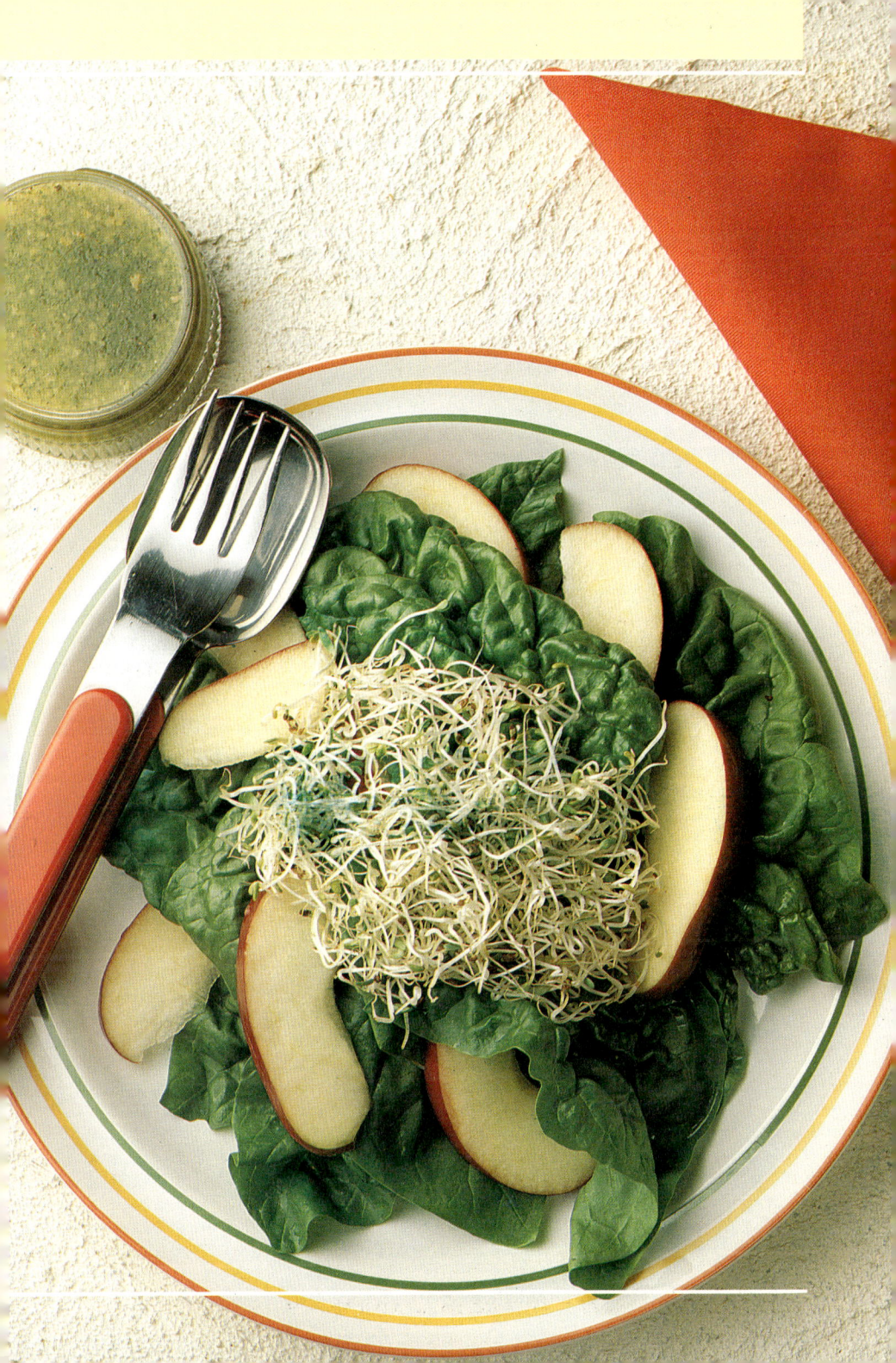

CUKE SALAD

Refreshing and crunchy, this low calorie salad provides a cool light accompaniment to a spicy or rich main course.

20cm cucumber
3 spring onions, finely
  sliced
1 Tbsp finely chopped
  root ginger

¼ cup spiced vinegar
1 tsp sugar
freshly ground black
  pepper

Peel the cucumber if the skin is bitter, slice finely. Mix the cucumber, spring onions, ginger, vinegar, sugar and pepper together. Refrigerate 1 hour before serving.
Serves 4 [62 kJ (15 Cal) per serve].

TABBOULEH

This traditional Lebanese salad uses wheat — a low fat, high fibre grain, which is also a valuable source of B vitamins, iron and calcium

1½ cups bulgur wheat
  (cracked wheat)
3 tomatoes
¼ cup sunflower seeds
½ cup finely chopped
  fresh parsley
¼ cup finely chopped
  fresh mint

2 Tbsp spiced vinegar
1 Tbsp polyunsaturated
  oil
½ tsp brown sugar
freshly ground black
  pepper

Place the wheat in a bowl and cover with boiling water. Stand 30 minutes. Rinse with cold water and drain well. Cut each tomato into wedges. Place the wheat, tomatoes, sunflower seeds, parsley and mint in a bowl. Mix the vinegar, oil, brown sugar and pepper together. Pour over the wheat mixture. Mix well.
Serves 6 [721 kJ (172 Cal) per serve].

Photograph page 159

50:50 RICE SALAD

Rice, especially brown varieties, is high in fibre and B vitamins, providing some protein as well. Easily prepared, it mixes well with dried fruit, giving an interesting texture and flavour.

½ cup brown rice
½ cup white rice
¼ cup roughly chopped crystallised ginger
¼ cup roughly chopped dates

2 Tbsp finely chopped fresh mint
1 Tbsp vinegar
1 Tbsp soy sauce
1 tsp sugar

Place the brown rice in boiling water and boil 20 minutes. Add the white rice and continue boiling for 15 minutes or until the white rice is tender and the brown rice is slightly chewy. Add extra boiling water if necessary. Rinse under cold running water and drain well. Cool. Mix the rice, ginger, dates, mint, vinegar, soy sauce and sugar together. Serves 4 [650 kJ (155 Cal) per serve].

Variation: Dried apricots and figs may be substituted for the ginger and dates.

Microwave
Place the brown rice and 3 cups cold water in a large, microwave proof bowl. Cover and cook on 100% power for 12 minutes. Add the white rice and cook on 100% power for a further 12 minutes or until the white rice is tender and the brown rice slightly chewy.

BEAN SALAD

This salad, high in fibre and rich in B vitamins, offers a variety of flavours and textures. Take care not to overcook the beans, otherwise they become soft and mushy.

1 cup mixed dried beans
1 onion, finely chopped
1 tsp finely chopped root ginger
½ cup sliced celery
1 cup cauliflower florets

1 carrot, finely sliced
½ green pepper, finely diced
¾ cup white wine vinegar
¼ cup sugar
1 cup water

Soak the beans overnight in water. Drain. Bring them to the boil in fresh water and simmer 45-60 minutes or until the beans are soft. Drain. Combine the beans, onion, ginger, celery, cauliflower, carrot and green pepper. In a small saucepan heat the vinegar, sugar and water, stir until the sugar is dissolved. Cool and pour over the bean mixture. Refrigerate 1-2 hours before serving.
Serves 6 [716 kJ (171 Cal) per serve].

Microwave
Place the soaked beans in boiling water and cook on 100% power for 20 minutes or until the beans are soft. Stand 10 minutes. Drain. In a microwave proof bowl combine the vinegar, sugar and water. Cook on 100% power for 1½-2 minutes. Stir once during cooking. Cool and pour over the bean mixture.

Photograph opposite page

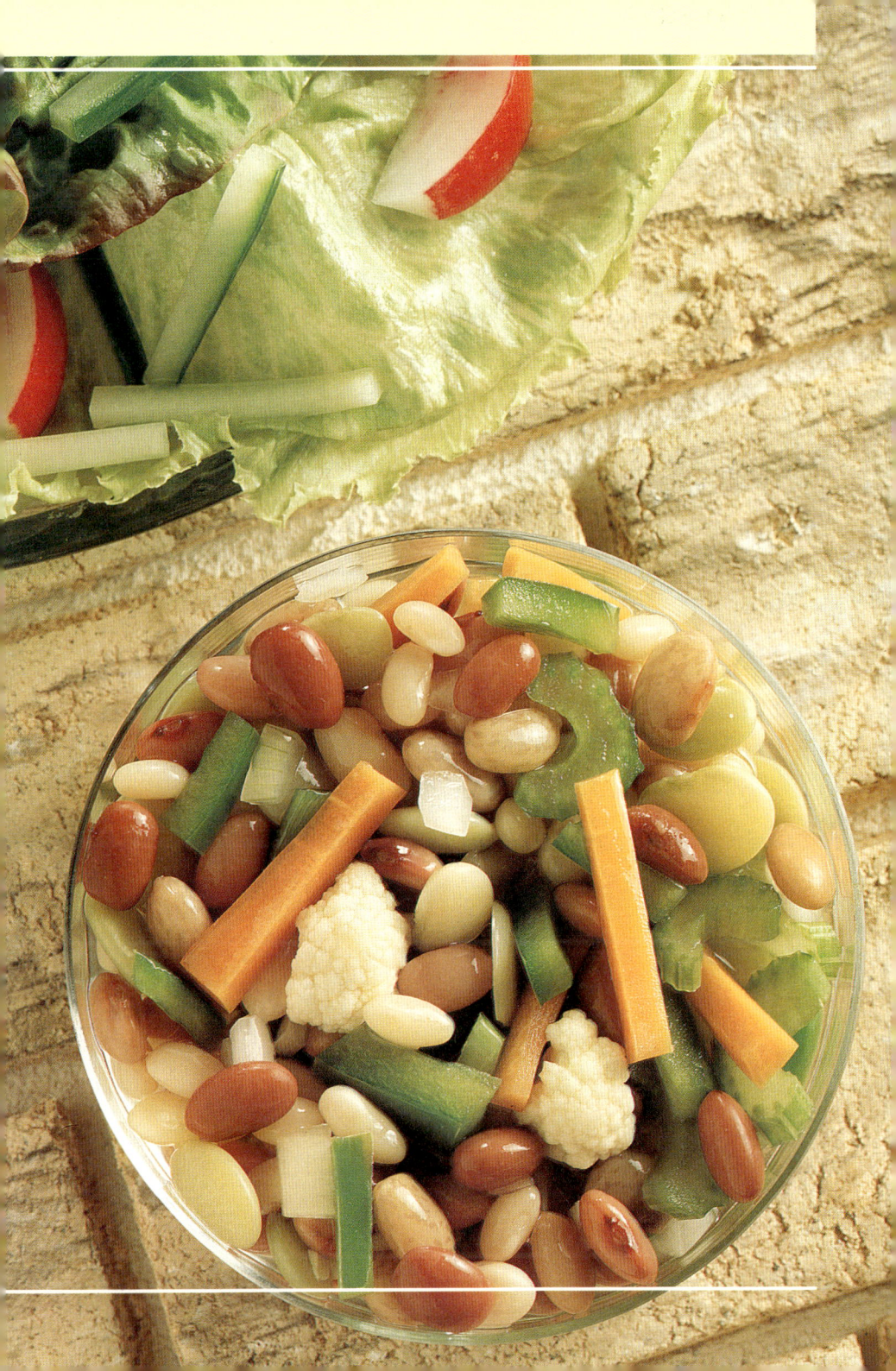

GARDEN GREEN SALAD WITH CREAMY DRESSING

This is a creamy low fat salad dressing which provides a low fat alternative to the mayonnaise and condensed milk dressings.

Make the most of the large variety of salad greens available such as different lettuce types, (cos, butterhead, iceberg, red lettuce), endive, watercress, celery leaves, spinach, silverbeet, bean sprouts, alfalfa sprouts, witloof.

Tear leafy greens into bite-sized pieces.
Toss all salad ingredients together in a large bowl.
Serve dressing separately.

Creamy Dressing

1 cup natural low fat yoghurt
½ tsp prepared mustard

freshly ground black pepper
1 Tbsp finely chopped fresh parsley or chives

Mix the yoghurt, mustard, pepper and parsley together.
[546 kJ (130 Cal) per recipe].

Photograph page 127

WINTER SLAW

A low fat yoghurt dressing can increase the protein content of a salad. This recipe combines yoghurt with fruit juice to add a little tang and extra vitamin C.

3 cups finely shredded
  cabbage
1 cup finely sliced
  celery

1 cup mandarin
  segments
¼ cup finely chopped
  fresh parsley

Mandarin Dressing

¼ cup natural low fat
  yoghurt
2 Tbsp mandarin juice

½ tsp grated mandarin
  rind
½ tsp dry mustard

Combine the cabbage, celery, mandarin, parsley and mandarin dressing.

Mandarin Dressing
Blend the yoghurt, mandarin juice, mandarin rind and mustard together.
Serves 6 [196 kJ (47 Cal) per serve].

Variation: Try oranges or tangelos in place of the mandarins.

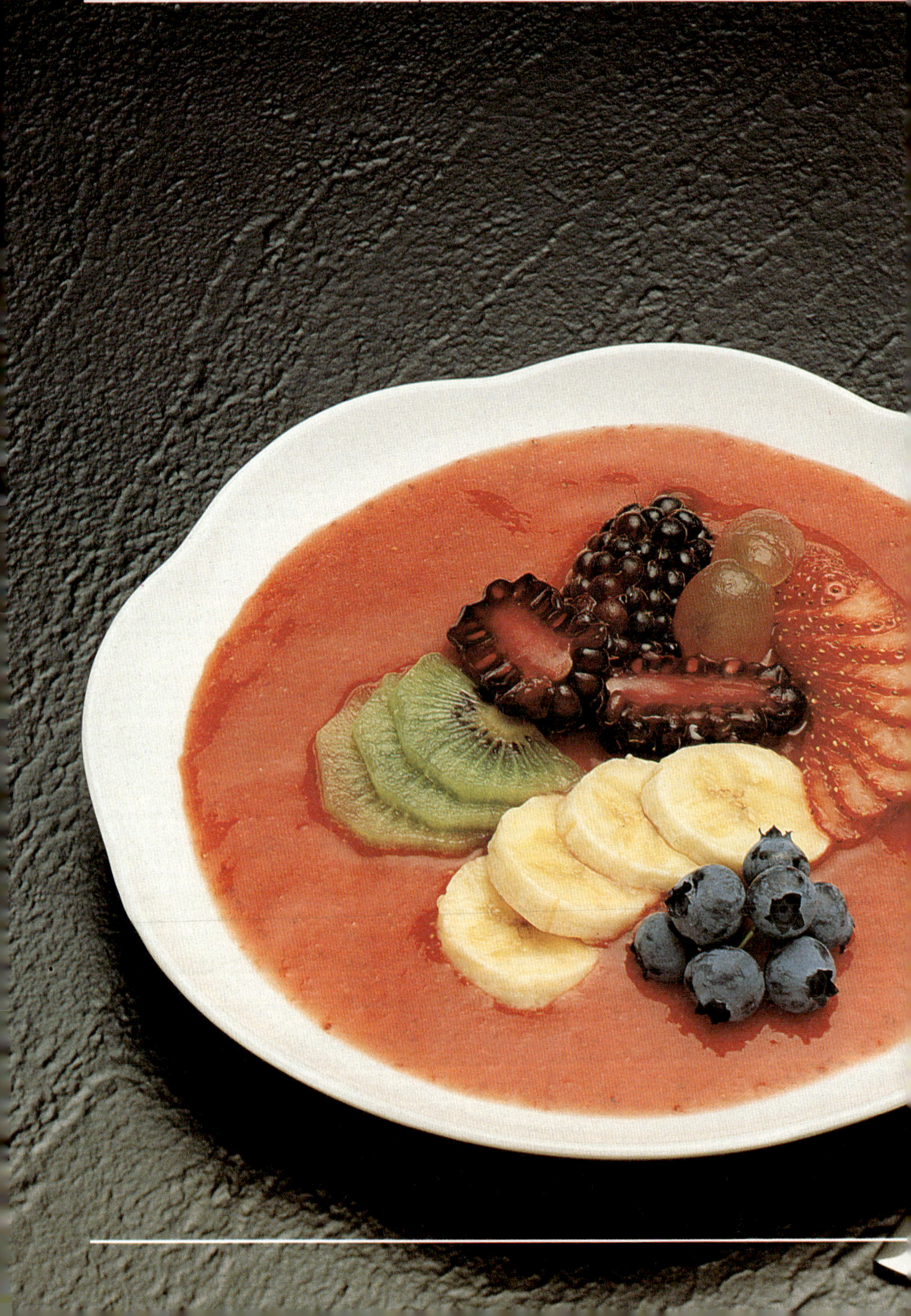

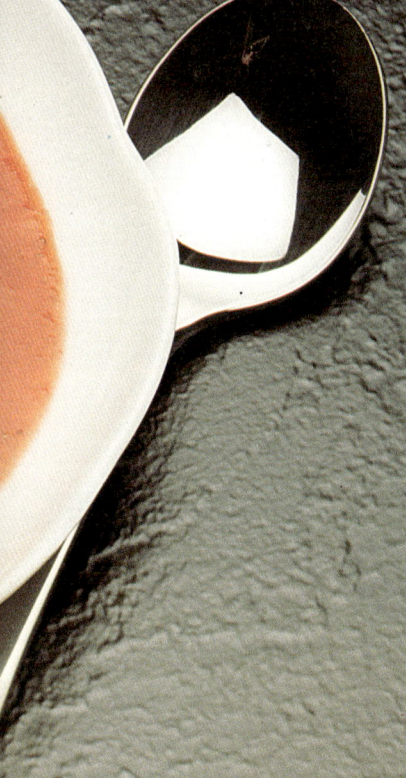

DESSERTS

Following the trend away from rich and stodgy puddings the recipes that follow are simple and wholesome. Included may be some of your old family favourites, slightly modified but tasting just as good. Many are based on fresh fruit in season — always an economical and nutritious way to end a meal.

Photograph: Arranged Fruit Salad (p.132).

ARRANGED FRUIT SALAD

Fresh seasonal fruit is a good source of vitamins, minerals and fibre — a colourful and refreshing end to any meal.

2 cups fresh strawberries
4 cups selected seasonal fruit such as:— blueberries, boysenberries, raspberries, strawberries, or grapes; slices of banana, kiwifruit, tamarillo, orange or mandarin;wedges of apricot, peach, apple or pear

Puree the strawberries and pour onto 4 flat luncheon plates. Arrange the selected fruit decoratively on top.
Serves 4 [410 kJ (98 Cal) per serve].,

Variation: Frozen berryfruit may be used in place of the fresh strawberries. Thaw 400 g of fruit and process until smooth. Adjust sweetness if necessary with 1-2 Tbsp sugar.

Photograph page 130

BAKED APPLES

Apples provide a good source of vitamins and fibre — especially in the skin. The different dried fruits and nuts in the fillings offer a variety of flavours — as well as adding extra fibre and minerals.

4 medium apples
½ cup natural low fat yoghurt

Core the apples. Fill with the chosen filling. Bake covered at 180° C for 30 minutes, or until the apples are softened. Reserve 3 Tbsp of the cooking juices. Mix with the yoghurt. Serve as a sauce with the apples.
Serves 4 [Apricot 581 kJ (138 Cal) per serve],
[Walnut 960 kJ (229 Cal) per serve],
[Banana 512 kJ (122 Cal) per serve].

Microwave

Cook on 100% power for 7-8 minutes.
Stand 4 minutes.

Apricot Filling

¾ cup finely chopped
  dried apricots
¼ cup natural low fat
  yoghurt

¼ tsp freshly grated
  nutmeg

Mix the apricots, yoghurt and nutmeg together.

Walnut and Date Filling

½ cup finely chopped
  walnuts
¾ cup finely chopped
  dates

1 tsp grated lemon rind
1 Tbsp lemon juice

Mix the walnuts, dates, lemon rind and juice
to a paste.

Banana and Orange Filling

1 large banana
2 tsp grated orange rind

1 Tbsp bran
2 Tbsp currants

Mash the banana. Mix the banana, orange rind,
bran and currants together.

FRUIT WHIP

A deliciously simple way of bringing out the best in fruit. Light and airy and fat free. Make the most of fruit in season for an economical dessert.

1 Tbsp gelatine
½ cup boiling water
1 Tbsp lemon juice

1 cup fruit puree
  (eg: apricot, peach, berryfruit)
2 egg whites
2 Tbsp sugar

Sprinkle gelatine over the water and stir until dissolved. Cool, then blend in the lemon juice and fruit puree. Chill until the mixture is slightly thickened. Beat the egg whites until soft peaks form. Add the sugar gradually and continue beating until firm peaks stand up when beater is removed. Beat gelatine mixture until light and doubled in volume. Fold into the egg white mixture. Spoon into a 4 cup capacity serving dish or 6 individual dishes.
Serves 6 [278 kJ (66 Cal) per serve].

Cover photograph

TAMARILLO TURNOVER

Tamarillos are tangy, richly red and high in vitamin C. To keep the calories down in this recipe, the pastry has been used only on the base. Wholemeal flour adds more fibre and flavour.

¾ cup flour
1 tsp baking powder
1 Tbsp icing sugar
¼ cup wholemeal flour
¼ cup polyunsaturated
  margarine

2-3 Tbsp cold water
1 cup peeled and
  grated apple
3-4 tamarillos, peeled
  and sliced
2 Tbsp brown sugar

Sift the flour, baking powder and icing sugar. Add the wholemeal flour and rub in the margarine until the mixture resembles fine breadcrumbs. Add enough water to form a dough. Roll out to a 22 cm square. Place in a 20 cm diameter flan dish. Spread the apples and tamarillos on top. Sprinkle with the brown sugar. Fold the corners of the base over the filling. Bake at 200°C for 20-25 minutes or until golden brown.
Serves 4 [1419 kJ (338 Cal) per serve].

RHUBARB AND GINGER CRUMBLE

A family favourite for cold winter nights. This recipe is a variation on the traditional crumble, with bran for extra fibre. Ginger gives a change in flavour.

3 cups chopped
   rhubarb
¼ cup water
1 Tbsp sugar
¼ cup roughly
   chopped crystallised
   ginger

¼ cup polyunsaturated
   margarine
¼ cup bran
¼ cup sugar
½ tsp ground ginger
½ cup wholemeal flour

Place the rhubarb and water in an ovenproof dish. Sprinkle over the first measure of sugar and the crystallised ginger. Blend the margarine, bran, second measure of sugar, ground ginger and wholemeal flour together. Sprinkle over the rhubarb. Bake at 180°C for 25-30 minutes or until golden brown.
Serves 4 [1527 kJ (364 Cal) per serve].

Microwave
Cover and cook the rhubarb, water, first measure of sugar and ginger on 100% power for 4 minutes. Add the topping and cook on 100% power for 2 minutes. Grill for 3-5 minutes if wished.

MULLED PEARS

Sure to impress your guests, this light dessert will finish off a more substantial meal. The arrangement of fruit on the plate is not difficult.

½ cup red wine
2 Tbsp sugar
pinch ground
   cinnamon (optional)

½ cup water
2 pears, peeled

Place the red wine, sugar, cinnamon and water in a small saucepan. Heat, stirring until the sugar dissolves. Add the pears. Cover and simmer 15-20 minutes or until the pears are tender. Remove the pears and reduce the syrup by boiling to a thick consistency. Cut the pears in half lengthwise and remove the cores. Place pear halves cut side down on a board. Cut slices 1cm wide, starting 2cms from the top of the pear and cutting to the base. Press pears gently to fan slices out. Pour the sauce onto each serving plate and place the pears on top. Serves 4 [411 kJ (98 Cal) per serve].

Microwave
Omit the water. Place the red wine, sugar and cinnamon in a microwave proof dish. Cook on 100% power for 1 minute. Stir to dissolve the sugar. Add the pears. Cover and cook on 100% power for 7-8 minutes. Stand 8 minutes. Remove the pears and prepare as instructed. Mix 1 Tbsp of cornflour and 1 Tbsp of water to a paste. Add to the sauce. Cook on 100% power for 3-4 minutes or until thickened. Serve as instructed.

Photograph opposite page

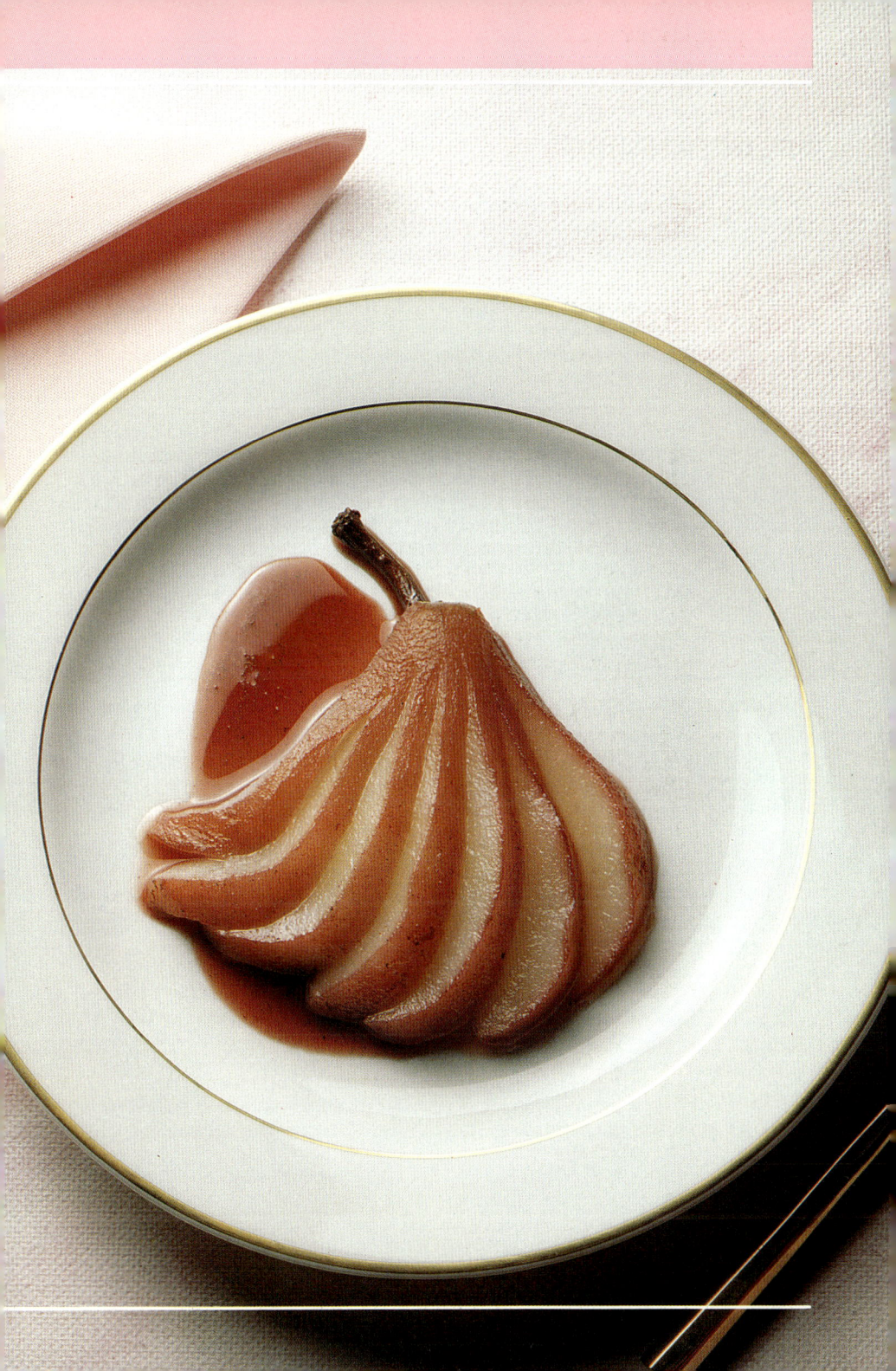

FRUIT SORBET

A very light refreshing dessert to finish off a substantial meal. Experiment with different varieties of fruit in season.

1 cup water
½ cup sugar
1 cup thin fruit puree
   (eg: tamarillos,
   berryfruit, stonefruit)

2 Tbsp lemon juice
1 egg white

Boil the water and sugar together for 5 minutes, cool and add the fruit puree and lemon juice. Mix thoroughly and pour into a 15 x 30cm freezing tray. Freeze for 1 hour. Beat the egg white until stiff. Turn the frozen mixture into a bowl and beat until light and fluffy. Fold the egg white into the frozen mixture and lightly mix. Freeze for 2-3 hours or until solid. Serves 4[764 kJ (182 Cal) per serve].

CARAMELISED ORANGES

The natural flavour of oranges is heightened in this delicious yet simple dessert. Oranges are a rich source of vitamin C.

6 oranges
⅓ cup sugar

1 cup water

Using a potato peeler remove the rind from 2 oranges. Cut into very thin needleshreds. Place the sugar in a heavy based saucepan. Heat until the sugar turns a golden brown. Slowly and carefully add the water. Add the rind and simmer for 5 minutes. Remove the skin and pith from the oranges. Slice horizontally and remove all pips. Place in a bowl. Pour over the caramel sauce. Serve chilled.
Serves 6 [482 kJ (115 Cal) per serve].

Variation: As a special treat add 2-3 Tbsp of orange flavoured liqueur to the caramel sauce.

COFFEE BANANA PIE

Similar to a cheesecake, this pie is an example of how a sweet dish can still be good value, thanks to a minimal amount of both sugar and fat. The recipe uses low fat cheese, yoghurt and the whites only of the eggs.

¼ cup polyunsaturated margarine
1 cup digestive biscuit crumbs
1 Tbsp gelatine
¼ cup boiling water
1 cup natural low fat cottage cheese

½ cup natural low fat yoghurt
¼ cup honey
2 tsp instant coffee powder
2 egg whites
2 bananas
2 tsp brown sugar

Melt the margarine and mix in the biscuit crumbs. Press into the base of 22cm diameter dish and refrigerate until firm. Dissolve the gelatine in the water and cool. Blend the cottage cheese, yoghurt, honey and coffee powder until smooth. Beat the egg whites until stiff. Fold the gelatine and egg whites into the cottage cheese mixture and pour over the biscuit base. Refrigerate for 2-3 hours or until set. Peel the bananas and slice into rings. Place on the pie, sprinkle with the brown sugar. Serves 6 [1287 kJ (306 Cal) per serve].

APPLE CRACKERS

*Dried apricots are ideal partners for less sweet
fruits, providing good value (fibre and iron), colour
and sweetness. Thanks to the filo pastry this novel
dessert is low in fat as well.*

3 medium apples,
  peeled and chopped
½ cup finely chopped
  dried apricots
1 Tbsp brown sugar

½ tsp mixed spice
8 sheets filo pastry
¼ cup polyunsaturated
  oil
orange rind for garnish

Mix the apples, apricots, brown sugar and mixed
spice together. Lay one sheet of filo pastry on a
clean flat surface. Brush sparingly with the oil.
Cover with a second sheet of pastry. Cut in half
widthwise. Spoon one eighth of the fruit mixture
along one end of the pastry. Roll to form a tube.
Crumple the ends to form a cracker. Tie loosely
with string. Repeat with remaining filo pastry and
fruit filling. Bake at 200° C for 20 minutes or until
golden brown. Remove the string. Cut 16 long
strips of orange rind and use these to tie knots at
each end of the cracker. Serve hot.
Serves 8 [765 kJ (182 Cal) per serve].

Variation: Make one large strudel. Reduce the filo
pastry to 4 sheets and the oil to 2 tablespoons.
Follow instructions as for Chicken Strudel.

Photograph opposite page

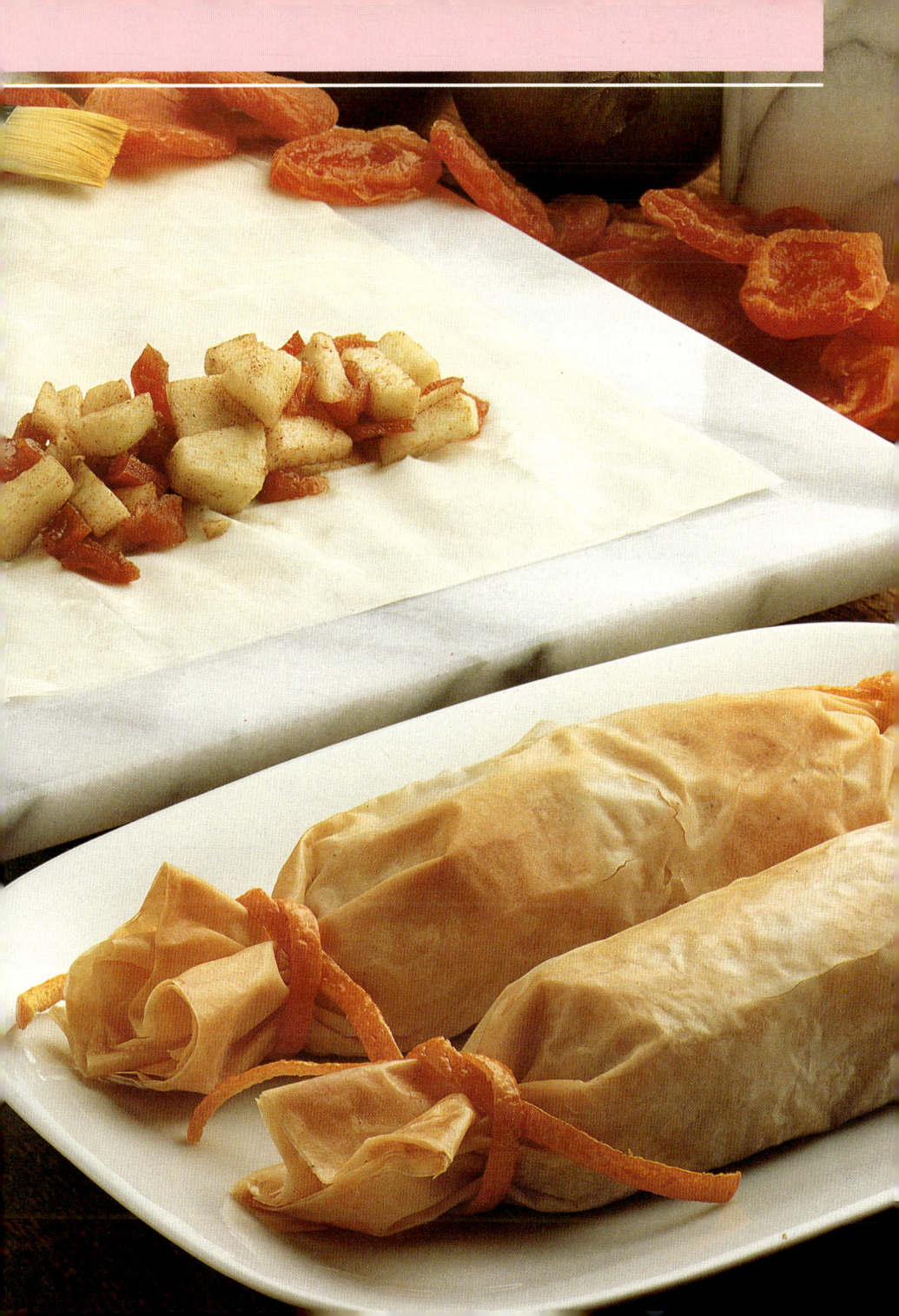

LEMON SPONGE PUDDING

A deliciously light pudding which is always a family favourite. Using non-fat milk and only the whites of eggs keeps the fat content down.

1 Tbsp polyunsaturated margarine	¼ cup lemon juice
	1 tsp grated lemon rind
½ cup brown sugar	1 cup non-fat milk
¼ cup flour	2 egg whites

Blend the margarine, brown sugar, flour, lemon juice and lemon rind together. Stir in the milk. Beat the egg whites until stiff and fold into the mixture. Pour into a lightly greased 20cm x 12cm baking dish. Place this dish in a roasting pan of hot water. Bake at 180°C for 40 minutes or until the custard is set and beginning to brown.
Serves 4 [824 kJ (196 Cal) per serve].

Variation: Use an orange in place of the lemon.

Microwave
Cover and bake on 70% power for 6-7 minutes. Stand 4 minutes. Grill for 3-5 minutes if wished.

FEIJOA AND RICE PUDDING

Milk puddings can be nutritious as well as delicious. Non-fat milk contributes little fat yet is still a good source of protein and calcium.

⅓ cup rice
2 Tbsp sugar

3 cups non-fat milk
1 cup peeled and
    chopped feijoas

Rinse and drain rice. Place the rice, sugar and milk in a 6 cup capacity baking dish. Bake at 150°C for 2-2½ hours or until the rice is tender. Stir frequently during cooking, adding extra milk if necessary. Lift the skin and fold in the feijoas.
Serves 4 [653 kJ (156 Cal) per serve].

Microwave
Cover and cook on 70% power for 25-30 minutes or until the rice is tender. Stand 15 minutes.
Add the feijoas and mix well.

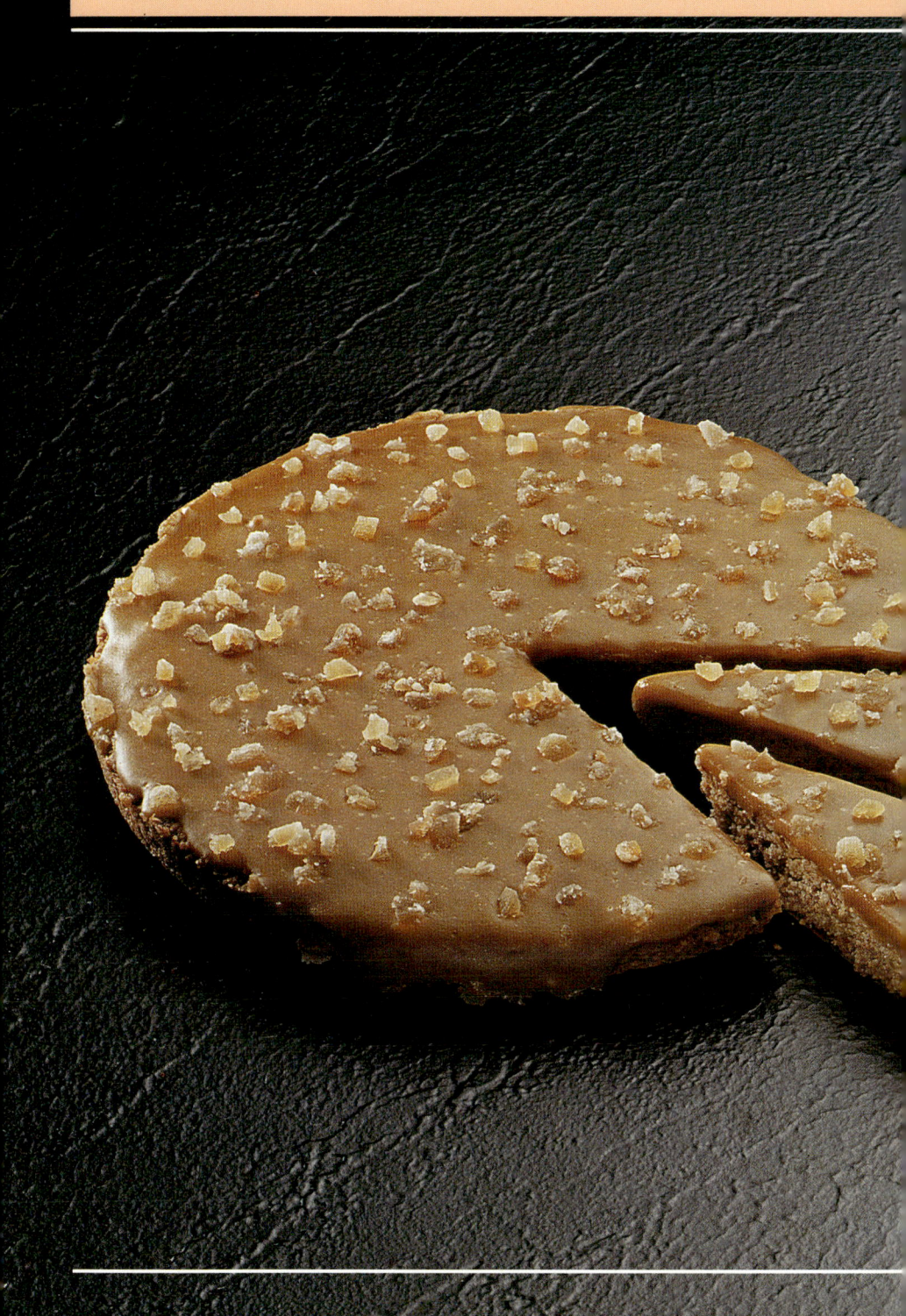

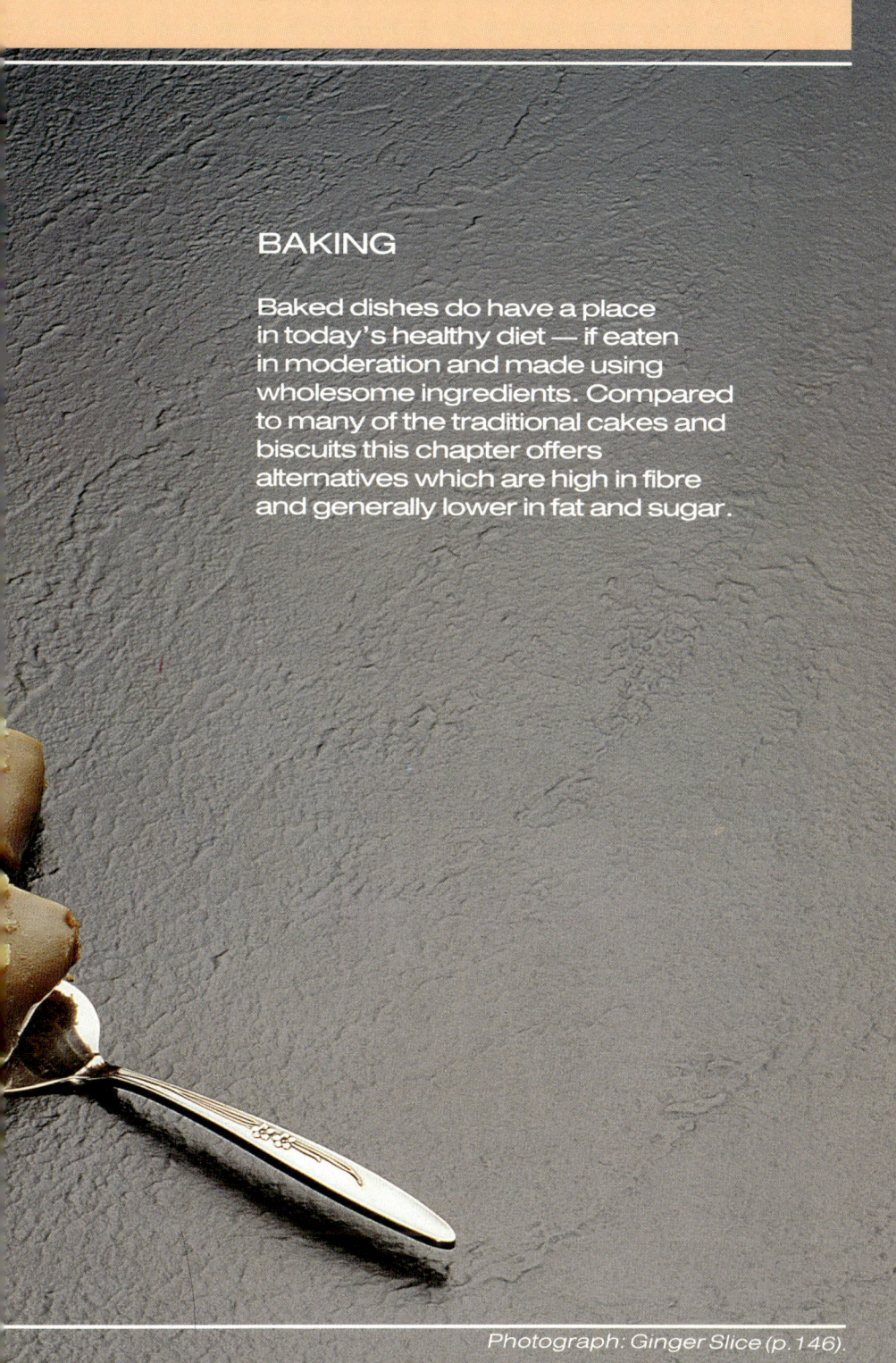

BAKING

Baked dishes do have a place
in today's healthy diet — if eaten
in moderation and made using
wholesome ingredients. Compared
to many of the traditional cakes and
biscuits this chapter offers
alternatives which are high in fibre
and generally lower in fat and sugar.

Photograph: Ginger Slice (p.146).

GINGER SLICE

This traditional slice is not especially low in sugar, but is low in fat. Wholemeal flour adds more fibre than found in the conventional version.

½ cup polyunsaturated
   margarine
⅓ cup sugar
1 cup wholemeal flour
½ cup rolled oats

1 tsp baking powder
1 tsp ground ginger
2 Tbsp chopped
   crystallised ginger
1 Tbsp chopped
   crystallised ginger

Ginger Topping

2 Tbsp polyunsaturated
   margarine
2 Tbsp golden syrup

½ cup icing sugar
1 tsp ground ginger

Cream the margarine and sugar until light and fluffy. Add the wholemeal flour, rolled oats, baking powder, ground ginger and first measure of crystallised ginger. Mix well. Press into lightly greased 25cm diameter or 28 x 18cm swiss roll tin. Bake at 180°C for 15-20 minutes or until golden brown. Spread the ginger topping over the slice while still warm and sprinkle with the second measure of crystallised ginger. Cut into 24 squares or triangles.

Ginger Topping
Melt the margarine and golden syrup. Add the icing sugar and ground ginger. Mix well.
Makes 24 pieces [517 kJ (123 Cal) per piece].

Microwave
Elevate and cook the base on 100% power for 3½-4 minutes. Heat the margarine and golden syrup on 100% power for 30-40 seconds.

Photograph page 144

SCRUMBLE SLICE

Scrumptious as well as nutritious this slice is packed with fibre from oats and flour. The dried fruit adds even more fibre and important vitamins and minerals for good health.

Filling:
1 cup water
1½ cups raisins
½ cup chopped dates

1 Tbsp grated lemon rind
¼ cup brown sugar
2 Tbsp wholemeal flour

Crust:
½ cup polyunsaturated oil
1 cup wholemeal flour
¾ cup wheatgerm
½ cup brown sugar

1 cup rolled oats
1 tsp cinnamon
1 tsp baking powder
¼ cup non-fat milk

Place the water, raisins, dates, lemon rind, brown sugar and wholemeal flour in a saucepan. Simmer 5-10 minutes or until thickened.

Crust
Mix all the crust ingredients together. Press half the crust into a 28 x 18cm sponge roll tin. Spread with the filling and cover with remaining crust. Press lightly. Bake at 180° C for 30-35 minutes or until golden brown. Cut when cool.
Makes 24 pieces [687 kJ (164 Cal) per serve].

Microwave
Cover and cook the filling on 100% power for 4 minutes. Assemble as instructed in an 18 x 28cm microwave proof slice tray. Elevate and cook on 100% power for 5-6 minutes. Stand 5 minutes.

PUMPKIN CAKE

Pumpkin adds sweetness and moistness to this cake, giving it a rich flavour and a good texture. Try serving wedges warm with low fat yoghurt for a delicious dessert.

1 cup wholemeal flour
¼ cup cornflour
2 tsp baking powder
1 tsp ground nutmeg
¾ cup brown sugar
2 eggs

¼ cup polyunsaturated oil
1 cup cooked pumpkin puree
4 Tbsp water
icing sugar to dust (optional)

Place the wholemeal flour, cornflour, baking powder, nutmeg and brown sugar in a bowl. Mix well. Separate the eggs. Beat the egg yolks, oil, pumpkin and water together. Add to the dry ingredients. Beat the egg whites until stiff. Fold into the pumpkin and flour mixture. Turn into a greased 20cm diameter ring tin. Bake at 180°C for 40-50 minutes or until an inserted skewer comes out clean. Cool on a wire rack. Dust with icing sugar if wished.
[8921 kJ (2124 Cal) per cake.]

Microwave
Turn into a lined 20cm diameter microwave proof ring mould. Elevate and cook on 100% power for 7-7½ minutes or until dry to touch. Stand 4 minutes before turning out.

BANANA CAKE

A moist flavoursome cake that's simple to make.
Bananas are naturally sweet and high in fibre.

⅓ cup polyunsaturated
   margarine
¼ cup sugar
2 eggs
1 cup mashed banana
½ tsp baking soda

¼ cup non-fat milk
1 cup wholemeal flour
1 cup flour
2 tsp baking powder
icing sugar to dust
   (optional)

Cream the margarine and sugar until light and
fluffy. Add the eggs and beat well. Mix in the
banana. Dissolve the baking soda in the milk. Fold
in the dry ingredients and milk alternately. Turn into
lightly greased 20cm diameter cake tin. Bake at
180°C for 45-55 minutes or until golden brown and
an inserted skewer comes out clean. Cool on a
wire rack. Dust with icing sugar if wished.
[9557 kJ (2276 Cal) per cake.]

Microwave
Increase the milk by 1 tablespoon. Turn into a
lined 20cm diameter microwave proof ring mould.
Elevate and cook on 100% power for 7½-8
minutes or until dry to touch.
Stand 4 minutes before turning out.

FRUITY BRAN LOAF

*A deliciously moist loaf that's easy to make —
packed with fibre and very low in fat. Best eaten the
day after baking.*

1½ cups All Bran
½ cup brown sugar
1½ cups mixed dried
   fruit (eg: sultanas,
   currants, raisins)

1½ cups non-fat milk
1 cup wholemeal flour
2 tsp baking powder

Soak the All Bran, brown sugar and dried fruit in
the milk for 30 minutes or until the milk has been
absorbed. Stir in flour and baking powder. Turn into
a lightly greased 17 x 10cm loaf tin. Bake at 180°C
for 1 hour or until golden brown and an inserted
skewer comes out clean.
Makes 1 Loaf [8224 kJ (1958 Cal) per loaf].

Microwave
Increase the milk to 1¾ cups. Elevate and cook in a
lined 19cm diameter microwave proof ring mould
on 100% power for 10-12 minutes or until the
surface is dry. Stand 5 minutes before turning out.

CUPPA SQUARE

*A quick and easy slice, full of fibre and low in fat.
The natural sweetness of the dried fruit helps to
keep the sugar low.*

1 cup bran
1 cup rolled oats
1 cup self raising
   wholemeal flour
½ cup raw sugar

1 cup roughly chopped
   walnuts
1 cup roughly chopped
   dried apricots
1 cup non-fat milk

Mix all the ingredients together. Press into a lightly
greased 18 x 28cm sponge roll tin. Bake at 150°C
for 25-30 minutes or until firm to touch.
Cut when cold.
Makes 24 pieces [543 kJ (129 Cal) per serve].

Photograph opposite page

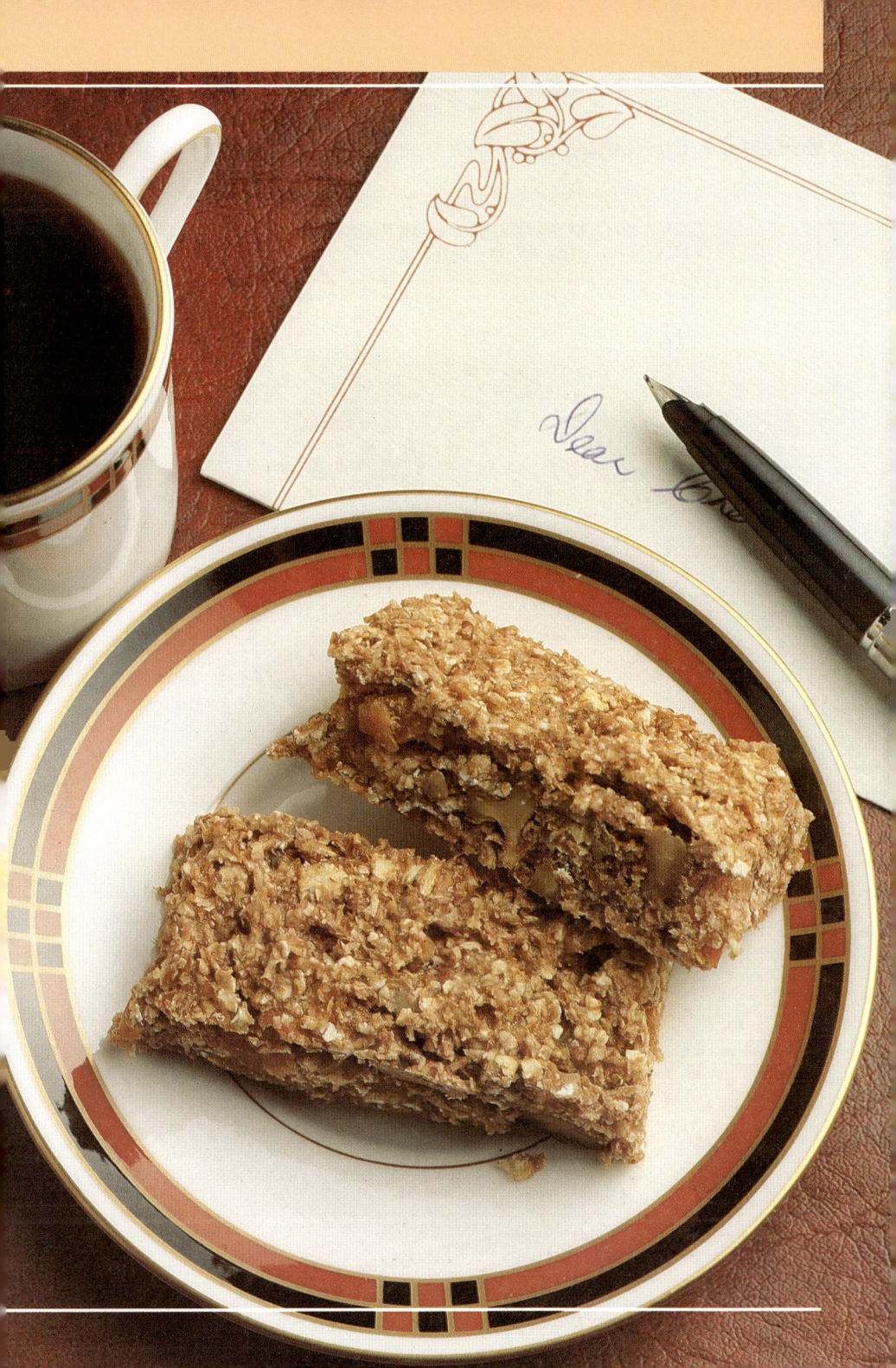

BRAN MUFFINS

A nutritious alternative to traditional cakes and biscuits. This recipe is very low in fat and offers a variety of flavours and textures. Enjoy them when fresh without being smothered with spreads.

1 cup wholemeal flour
2 cups bran
1 tsp baking powder
1½ tsp mixed spice
1 cup grated apple,
    skins on

½ cup non-fat milk
1 cup water
3 Tbsp golden syrup
1 tsp baking soda

Mix together the wholemeal flour, bran, baking powder, mixed spice and grated apple. Gently heat the milk, water and golden syrup. Stir in the baking soda. Pour the liquid ingredients into the dry ingredients and mix until just combined. Turn into lightly greased muffin tins. Bake at 200°C for 15-20 minutes or until golden brown.
Makes 1 dozen [430 kJ (102 Cal) per muffin].

Variations: In place of the apple and mixed spice try the following combinations:—

Blueberry: 1 cup blueberries, 1 tsp cinnamon

Citrus: 1 cup sultanas, 1 tsp grated orange rind

Carrot: 1 cup grated carrot, ½ cup toasted pumpkin seeds, ½ tsp ground nutmeg.

Microwave
Cook the milk, water and golden syrup on 100% power for 1 minute. Continue as above. Spoon the muffin mixture into a microwave proof muffin tray, lined with paper cases. Elevate and cook 5 muffins on 100% power for 2½-3 minutes or 6 muffins for 3½-4 minutes. Stand 4 minutes. Cook the next batch.

QUICK KIBBLED WHEAT BREAD

No need to knead with this recipe. Delicious homemade bread high in fibre and low in fat.

2½ cups warm water
2 tsp sugar
2 tsp dried yeast
2 cups flour

2 cups wholemeal flour
1 cup kibbled wheat
1 cup wheatgerm
1½ tsp salt

Mix the water and sugar together. Sprinkle with yeast. Stand in a warm place for 10-15 minutes or until frothy. In a large bowl mix together the flour, wholemeal flour, kibbled wheat, wheatgerm and salt. Pour in the yeast mixture and stir well. Turn into a well greased 10 cup capacity loaf tin. Stand in a warm place for 1½ hours or until the volume has doubled. Bake at 200°C for 40-50 minutes or until an inserted skewer comes out clean. Cover with foil for the first half of cooking.
Makes 1 loaf [12146 kJ (2892 Cal) per loaf].

CHEESE CRACKERS

Crisp biscuits are often difficult to make without a significant amount of fat. These crackers succeed with a minimum of fat from the cheese.

⅔ cup brown rice
75 g edam cheese
¼ cup natural low fat
  cottage cheese

¼ tsp paprika
2 Tbsp sesame seeds
paprika to sprinkle

Cook the brown rice in boiling water for 25-35 minutes or until tender. Drain. Place the cheese in a food processor fitted with a metal blade. Chop finely. Add the cottage cheese, brown rice and paprika. Pulse until evenly blended. Place teaspoonfuls on a non-stick baking tray or baking paper. Using wet fingers flatten to form circles 5cm in diameter. Sprinkle with sesame seeds and paprika. Bake at 180°C for 20-25 minutes or until golden brown and crisp. Cool on a wire rack. Store in an air tight container.
Makes 2 dozen [140 kJ (33 Cal) per biscuit].

Variation: This recipe makes a superb crust for a savoury flan or pie. Press into a 25 cm diameter loose bottomed or non-stick tin. Bake at 200°C for 30-40 minutes or until crispy. Delicious filled with Vegetable Curry (p 42).

Photograph opposite page

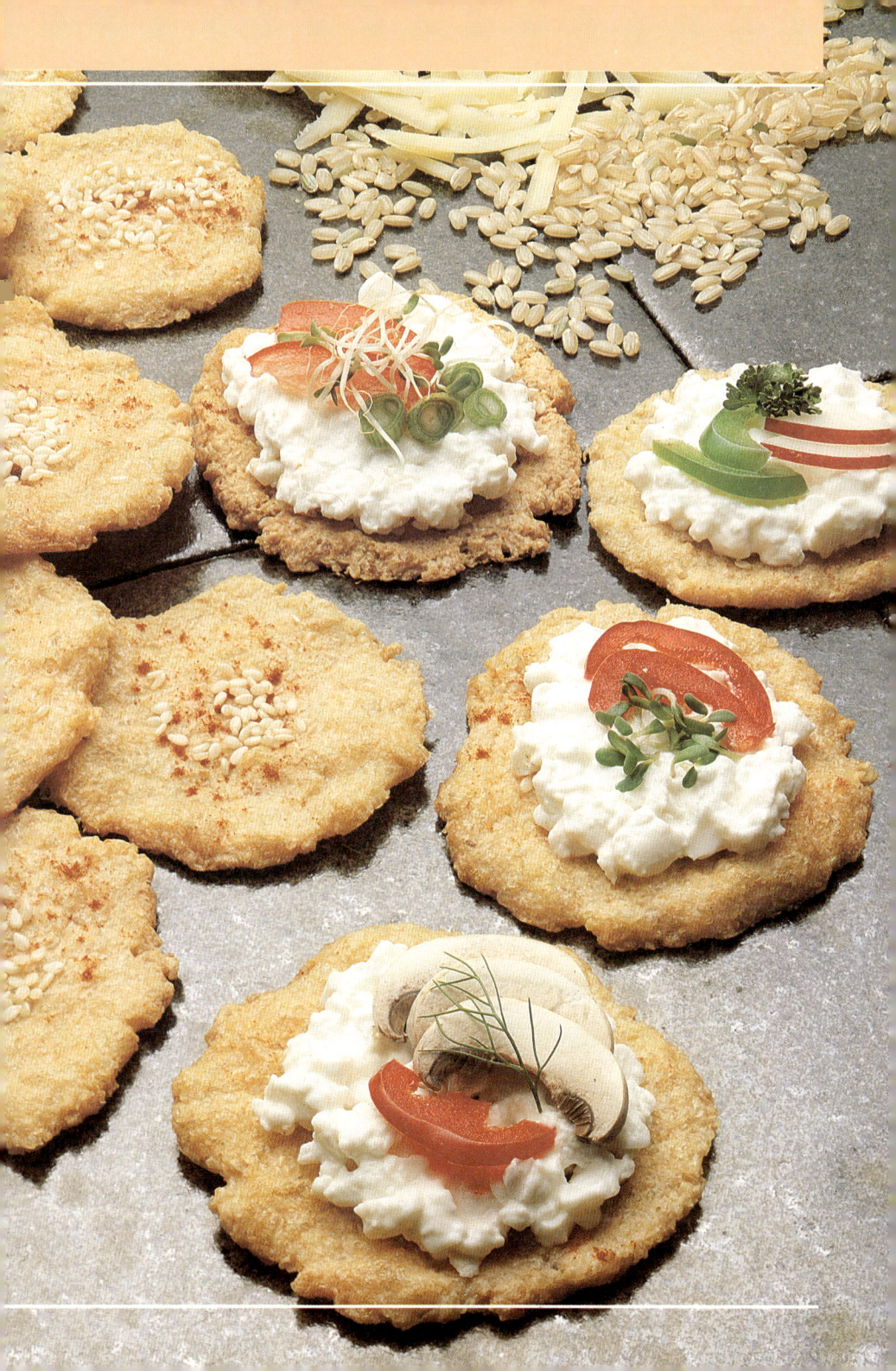

CARAWAY CRISPIES

The secret in making these is to roll the mixture as thinly as possible. These are crisp and tasty biscuits to serve with coffee or tea.

⅓ cup polyunsaturated
   oil
¼ cup brown sugar
2 eggs

2 cups wholemeal flour
2 tsp baking powder
½ cup bran
2 Tbsp caraway seeds

Beat the oil, brown sugar and eggs together until light and fluffy. Place the wholemeal flour, baking powder, bran and caraway seeds in a bowl. Add the egg mixture and mix to form a soft dough. Roll until very thin. Cut into squares. Place on a greased tray and bake at 180° C for 15 minutes or until golden brown.
Makes about 4 dozen [191 kJ (46 Cal) per biscuit].

OATY FRUIT BISCUITS

Using wholegrain oats for added fibre these biscuits also contain dried fruit which provides useful amounts of vitamins and minerals, as well as natural sweetness.

¼ cup polyunsaturated
   margarine
1 Tbsp golden syrup
1 egg, lightly beaten
1 cup wholegrain oats
1 cup wholemeal flour

1 tsp baking powder
¼ cup brown sugar
½ cup sultanas
½ tsp ground cloves

Melt the margarine and golden syrup. Mix all ingredients together. Roll spoonfuls of the mixture into balls and place on a lightly greased oven tray. Flatten. Bake at 180° C for 20-25 minutes or until golden brown.
Makes 2 dozen [383 kJ (91 Cal) per biscuit].

DATE SCONES

Scones are great when you're in a hurry. This recipe uses wholemeal flour for extra fibre and dried fruit for added sweetness. Don't just serve them for afternoon tea — use them in lunchboxes, picnics and light meals as well.

3 cups flour
2 Tbsp baking powder
1 cup wholemeal flour
3 Tbsp polyunsaturated
   oil

½ cup non-fat milk
¾ cup water
1 cup dates

Sift the flour and baking powder together. Add the wholemeal flour. Make a well in the centre, add the oil, milk and water. Mix to form a soft dough. Knead gently and roll out to a rectangle 26 x 40cm. Brush with cold water. Flatten the dates and place on half the scone dough. Fold the free half over and press down. Cut into 18 squares. Bake at 200°C for 10-15 minutes or until golden brown.
Makes 1½ dozen [615 kJ (146 Cal) per serve].

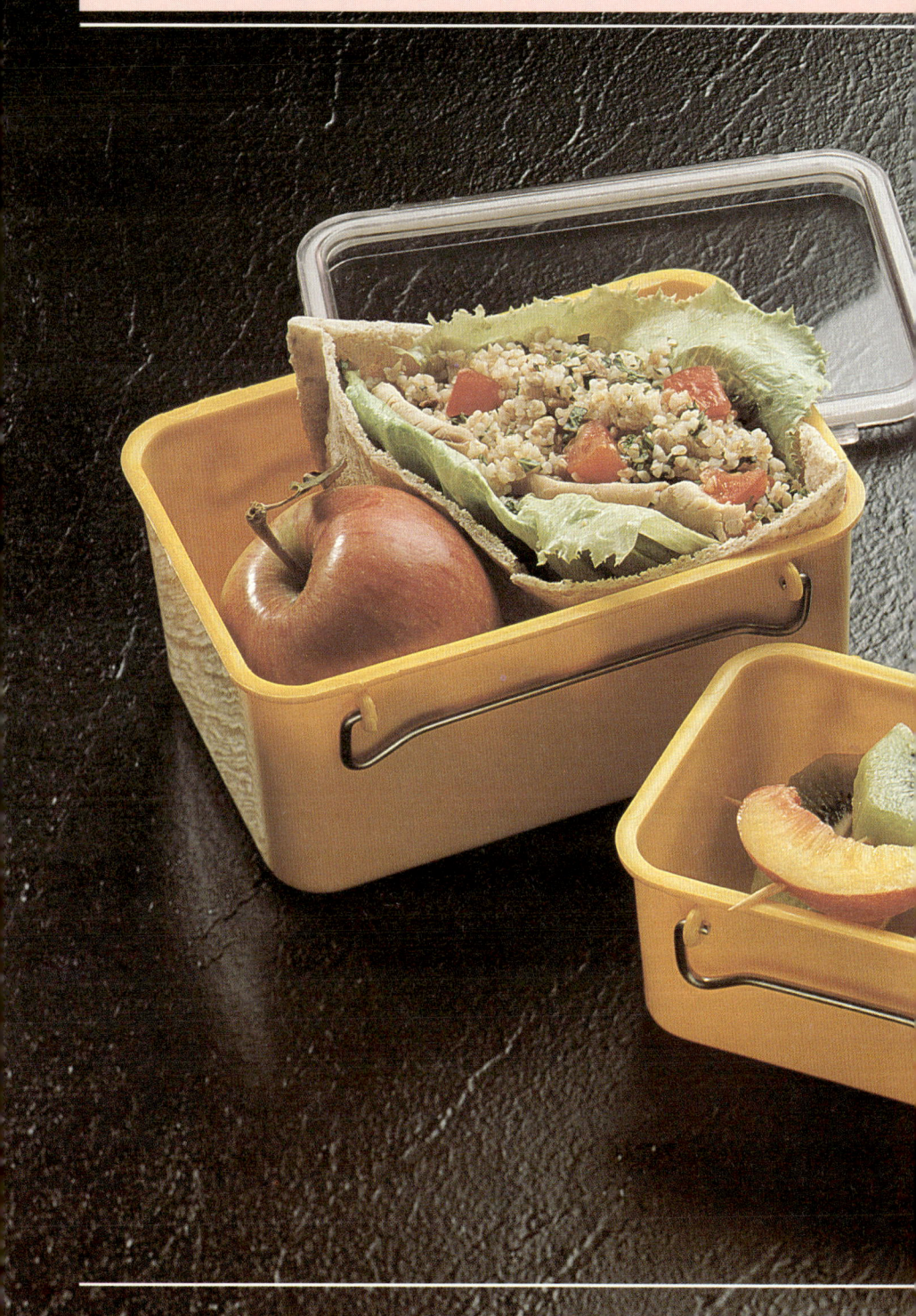

THE LUNCH BOX

There is often a problem of having
to constantly provide interesting and
nutritious packed lunches for school
and work. From super sandwiches
and savoury surprises to flask foods
and sweet treats to follow, this
chapter offers a range of varied and
tasty lunches sure to satisfy all the
family's lunchtime needs.

Photograph: Tabbouleh in Pita Bread (p. 124), Fruit Kebabs. (p. 170).

SCHOOL LUNCHES

Providing lunches which are interesting, varied and well balanced does take a little effort, but this time is well spent if it means the lunches are eaten and enjoyed — instead of ending up in the rubbish bin. A little surprise tucked into the children's lunch box makes lunchtime something to look forward to. Our suggestions which follow, take into account that time is often short when lunches are being prepared. It may be easier to give the children money to buy their lunch. This is fine as an occasional treat, but remember a school lunch is important — it should be just as substantial and well balanced as every other meal.

Photograph page 158

LUNCHES AT WORK

Working lunches vary so much — often just a bite on the run. Unfortunately there is not always a healthy choice available where and when you want it. But with a minimum of effort you can take a heart-healthy lunch from home every day. A lunch of sandwiches or rolls, accompanied by a piece of fresh fruit or fruit juice, can be an appetising and nutritious meal that will satisfy most people's needs. However, for more packed lunch suggestions refer to the ideas that follow.

SUPER SANDWICH

There are so many different combinations of breads, spreads, fillings and even shapes, that you could easily have a new and exciting sandwich every day of the year.

Bread
Vary the type of bread used:— wholemeal, wholegrain, rye, seed, white, pumpernickel, pita bread, french sticks, fruit loaves, rolls, buns or muffins. Even crackers or crispbreads offer a welcome change. For a delicious homemade bread try Quick Kibbled Wheat Bread (p 153).

Spreads
Polyunsaturated margarine spreads easily and should be used sparingly. Margarine is not always necessary if using a moist filling like cottage cheese or peanut butter (low salt).

Fillings
Here are some combinations to try . . .
1   Tuna, natural low fat cottage cheese and alfalfa sprouts.
2   Grated edam cheese, celery leaves and sliced tomato.
3   Natural low fat cottage cheese, finely chopped fresh mint and dates.
4   Sliced chicken, unsweetened crushed pineapple and lettuce.
5   Lean beef, thin apple slices and whole seed mustard.
6   Mashed banana, raisins and a sprinkling of lemon juice and cinnamon.
7   Grated carrot, bean sprouts and crunchy peanut butter (low salt).
8   Cucumber slices and finely chopped crabstick mixed with natural low fat yoghurt and chopped chives.

Shapes
Even the shape of a sandwich adds variety — they will taste the same but the change in shape adds eye appeal and interest.
Try
—   pinwheels using a mixture of brown and white bread
—   club sandwiches using a mixture of brown and white bread
—   the loaf sliced horizontally instead of vertically
—   long thin sandwiches — "soldiers"
—   cubes
—   triangles
—   dagwoods
—   open sandwiches
—   funny face sandwiches — for children arrange the salad vegetables to make a face on the bread.

Photograph page 165

SNAPPY SALADS

Enjoy salads year round by making the most of seasonal fruits and vegetables. See Chapter 8 on Salads for inspiration. When making your evening meal, make a little extra salad and pack it into a small container for lunch the next day. That, along with a roll and a piece of fruit is quick, easy and satisfying. Alternatively use the salad to fill a pita pocket.

FLASK FOOD

Flasks have revolutionised lunches — nothing beats piping hot soup on a cold winters day, or chilled soup in the heat of the summer. All our soups in Chapter 2 make delicious and filling lunchtime treats. The following recipes can be taken in wide-necked flasks to provide hot and hearty meals away from home.

Fish Ratatouille (p 59)
Smoked Hoki Pie (p 68)
Beef Stir-Fry (p 72)
Fruity Pork Stir-Fry (p 79)
Chilli Chicken (p 93)
Chicken and Vegetable Toss (p 100)
Chicken and Bean Hot Pot (p 96)
Stuffed Potatoes (p 54)
Stuffed Peppers (p 48)
Vegetable Curry (p 42)
Tofu and Vegetable Toss (p 52)

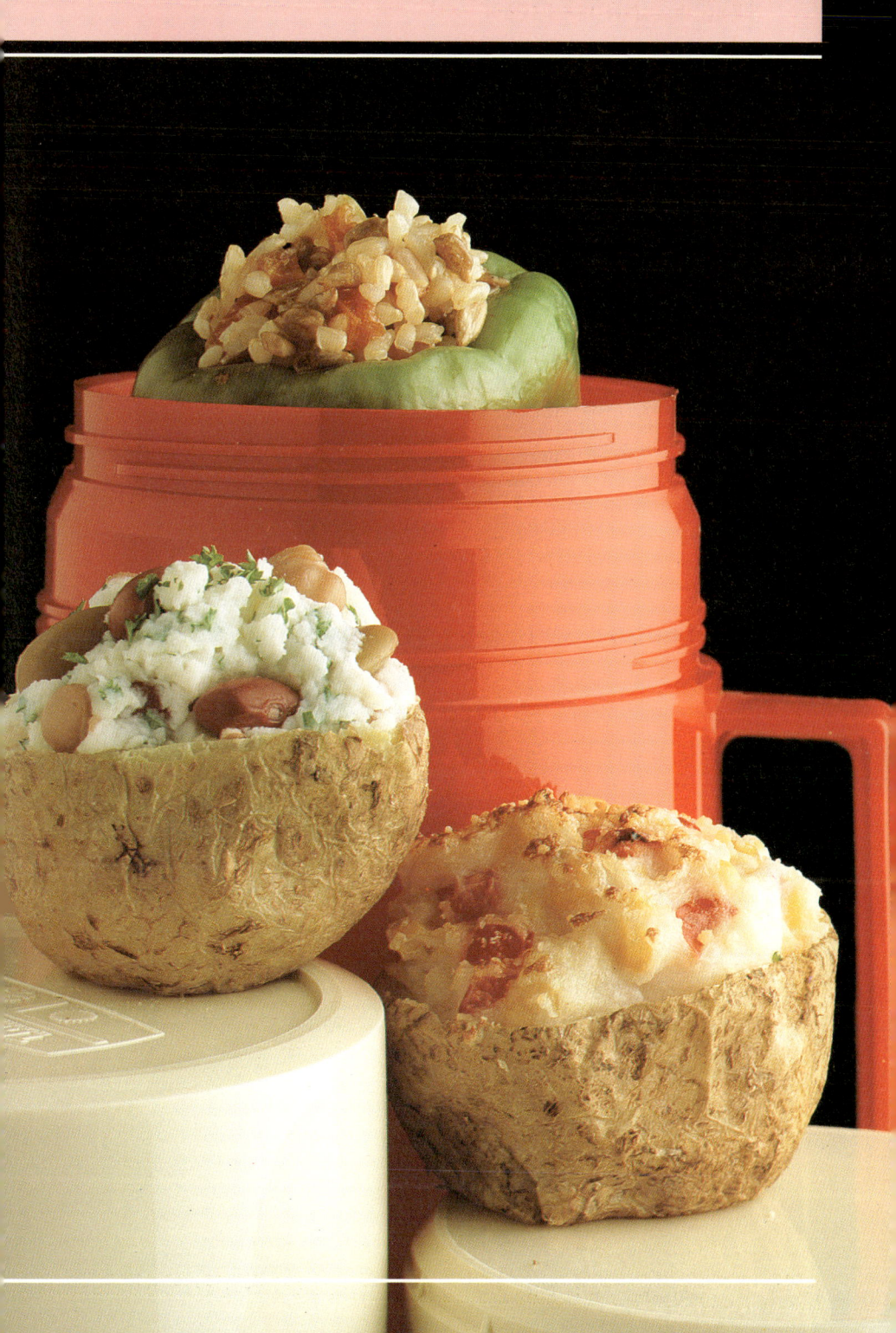

TASTY TREATS

The following savoury suggestions are fine served cold and travel well, offering interest and variety to lunchtime meals.

Celery sticks filled with Celery Dip (p 22) or Bacon and Garlic Dip (p 17)
Cheesey Bites (p 12) leave uncooked
Cheese Log (p 23) with crackers or as a filling for celery sticks
Chicken and Celery Loaf (p 92)
Sesame Chicken (p 102)
Tandoori Chicken (p 90)
Leek Filo Flan (p 41)
Carrot Loaf (p 50)
Pizza (p 47) — pita poppettes are especially suitable for children's lunches

SOMETHING SWEET WITH FRUIT TO FINISH

Many people like to finish a meal with something sweet. Mixed dried fruit and nuts are a good finishing off snack. Portable puddings such as fruit salads, fruit kebabs and yoghurt with added fresh fruit, also make a welcome change. Most people like to have a drink of some sort — select pure fruit juice or water in preference to fruit cordials or soft drinks. Those with a sweet tooth and who are not overweight may like to select a treat from Chapter 10 on Baking. Be sure to follow this with something crisp and crunchy, such as a piece of fresh fruit or slices of raw vegetables.

Photograph page 158

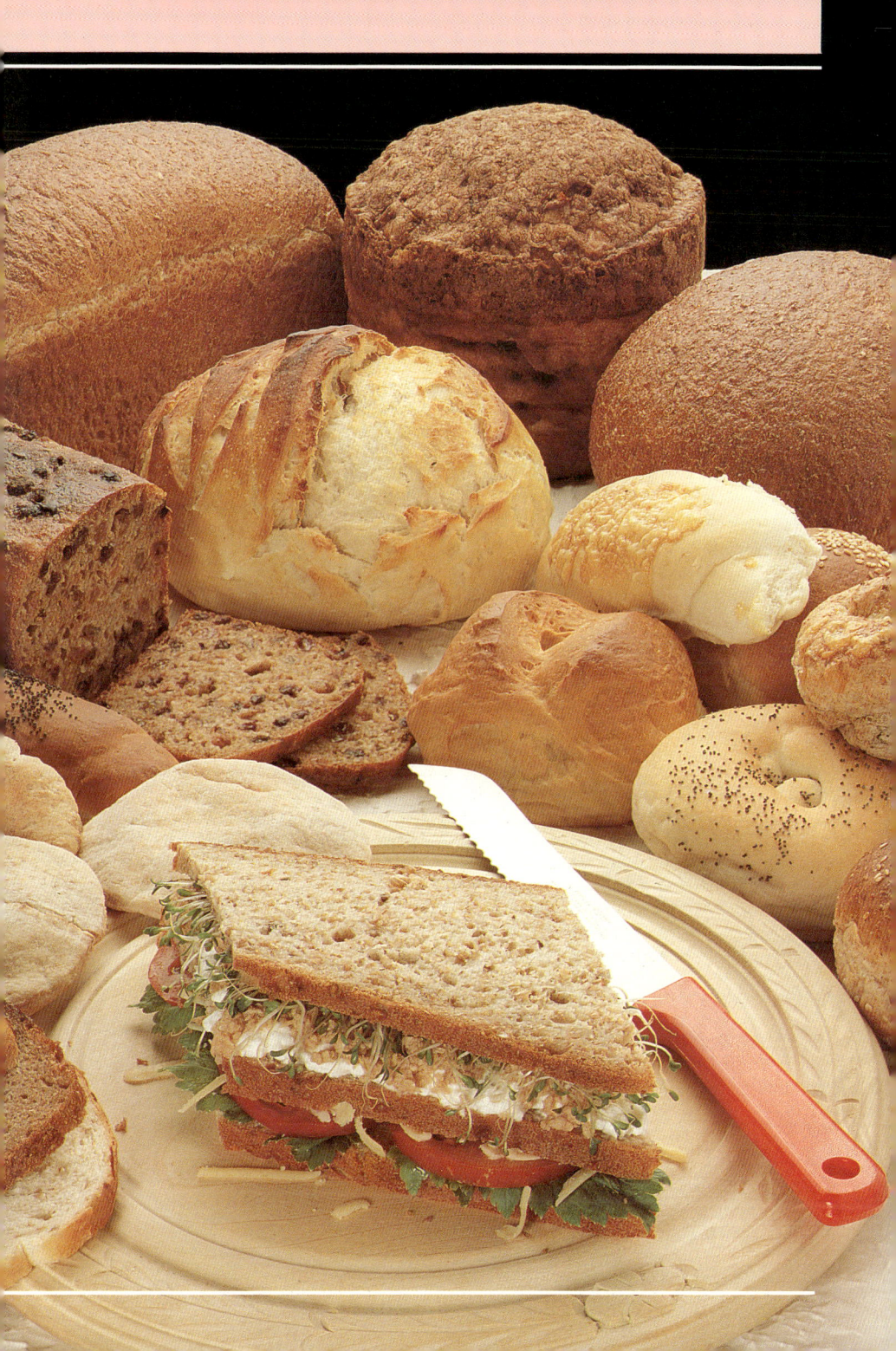

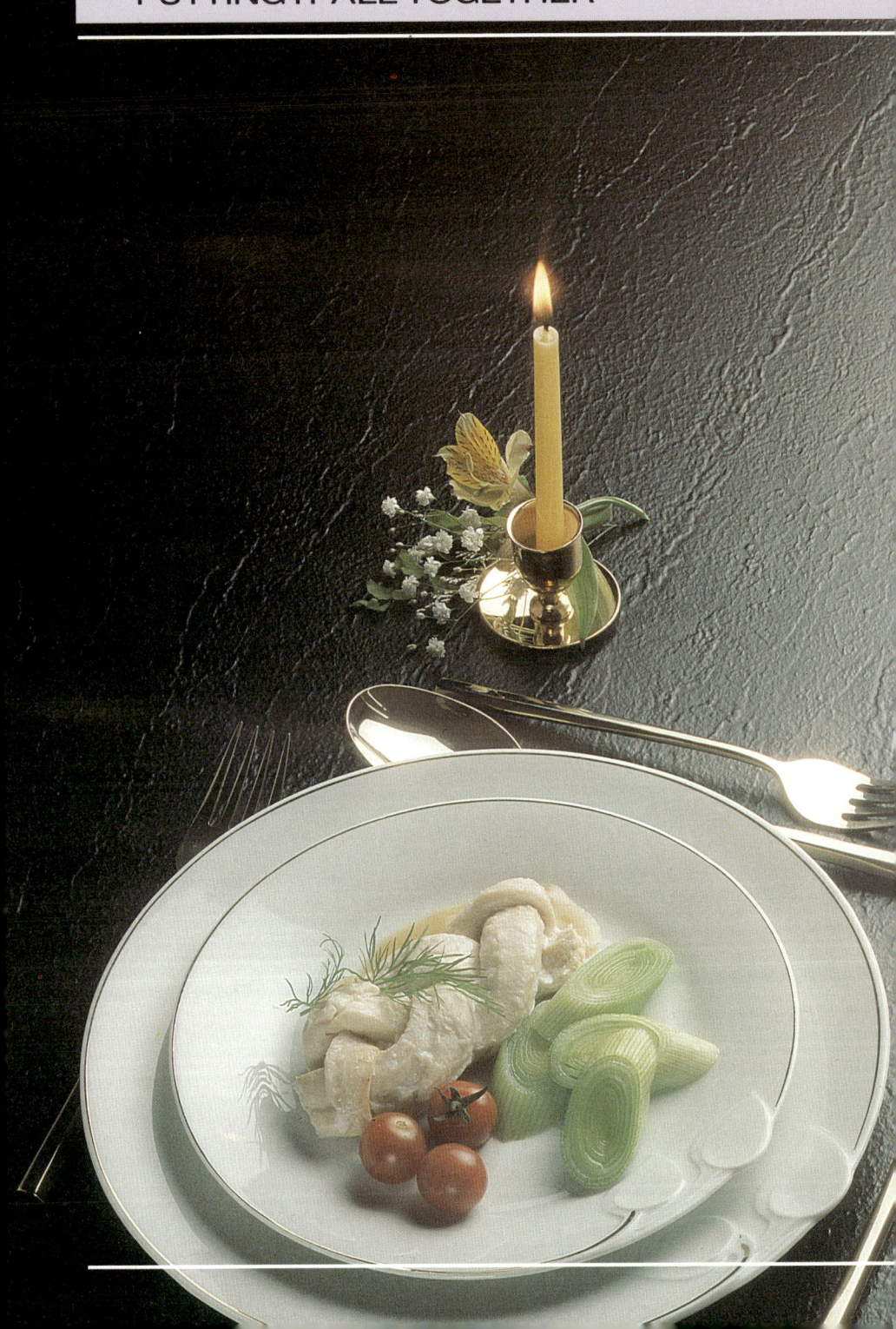

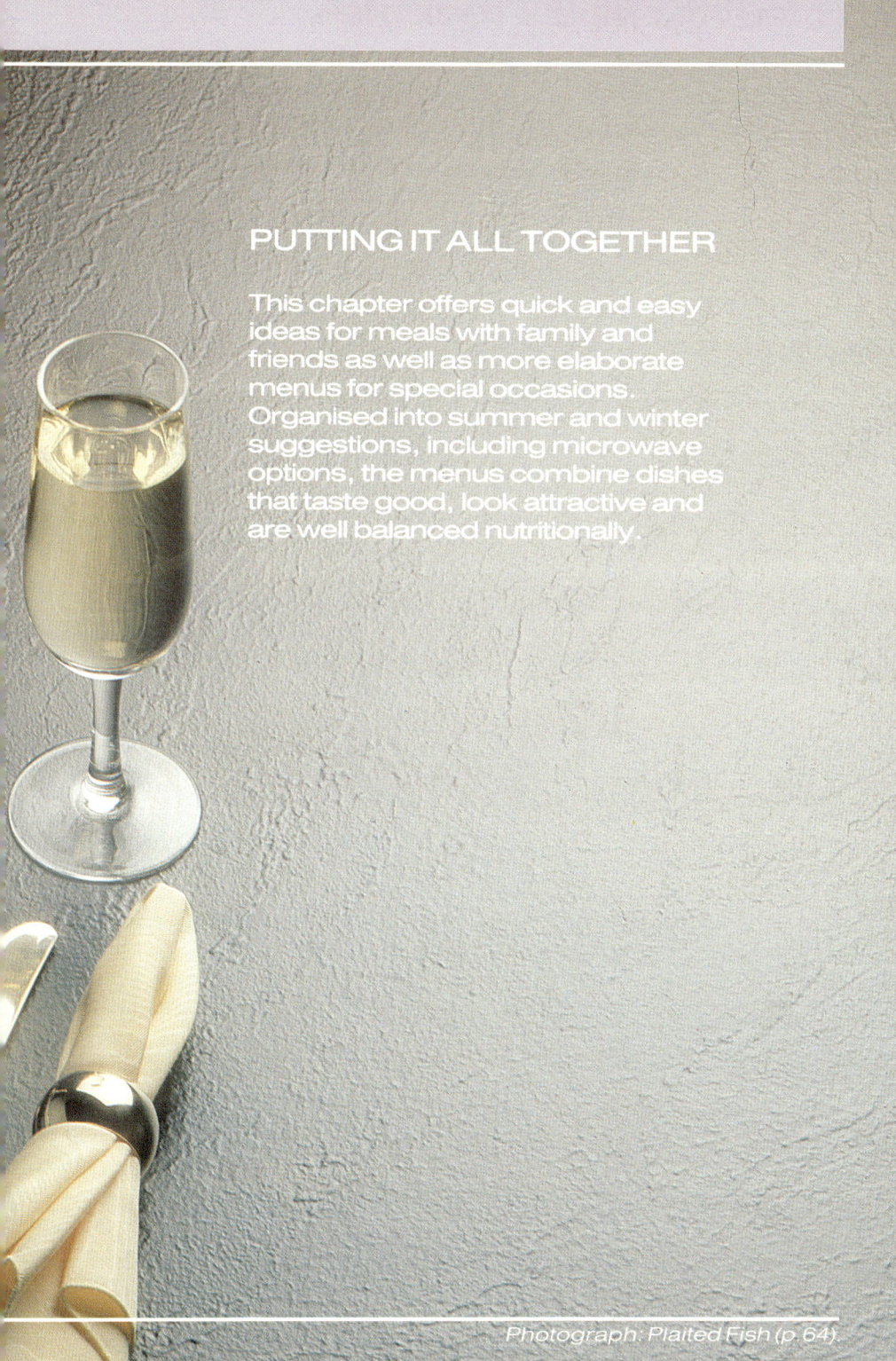

PUTTING IT ALL TOGETHER

This chapter offers quick and easy ideas for meals with family and friends as well as more elaborate menus for special occasions. Organised into summer and winter suggestions, including microwave options, the menus combine dishes that taste good, look attractive and are well balanced nutritionally.

Photograph: Plaited Fish (p 64).

FAMILY MEALS IN LESS THAN AN HOUR

Inspiration for easy and nourishing meals is often lacking at the end of a busy day. Select from our menus to suit your family's tastes.

Summer:

Menu One

Chilled Fruit Soup (p 34)
Italian Pasta (p 44)
Garden Green Salad (p 128)
Wholemeal Rolls

1 Prepare Italian Sauce.
2 Make Fruit Soup.
3 Prepare Green Salad.
4 Cook pasta.

Menu Two

Quick Corn Quiche (p 53)
Carrot and Poppyseed Salad (p 121)
Lettuce Salad
Mixed Grain Rolls
Fresh Fruit Salad

1 Prepare quiche.
2 Prepare Carrot and Poppyseed Salad.
3 Wash lettuce and tear leaves into bite-sized pieces.
4 Using seasonal fruit, prepare a fruit salad. Top with natural low fat yoghurt and chopped nuts if wished.

Menu Three — Using the Microwave

Chilli Bean Tacos (p 46)
Shredded Lettuce
Sliced Tomato
Grated Carrot
Grated Edam Cheese
Lemon Sponge Pudding (p 142)

1 Prepare the chilli bean mixture using a 310 g tin of kidney beans.
2 Shred the lettuce, slice the tomatoes and grate the carrot and cheese.
3 Prepare the lemon pudding. Serve hot or cold.
4 Heat the tacos and serve.

Winter:

Menu One

Beef Stir-Fry (p 72)
Rice
Rhubarb and Ginger Crumble (p 135)

1   Marinate the meat, reducing marinating time to 40 minutes.
2   Prepare rhubarb and ginger crumble.
3   Cook the rice.
4   Prepare vegetables for stir-fry.
5   Cook the stir-fry.

Menu Two

Minted Pea Soup (p 33)
Fish Souffle (p 69)
Nutty Brussels (p 110)
Tangy Carrots (p 114)

1   Prepare souffle.
2   Using frozen peas, prepare the soup.
3   Simmer the carrots.
4   Steam the Brussels sprouts.
5   Puree the soup.
6   Make the sauce for the carrots. Top the Brussels sprouts with nuts.

Menu Three — Using the Microwave

Lemon Chicken (p 97)
Baked Potatoes
Baked Pumpkin
Crispy Cabbage (p 110)
Banana Cake Wedges (p 149)

1   Cook the potatoes. Cover and stand.
2   Prepare the pumpkin into serving portions. Cook and stand.
3   Prepare and cook the chicken.
4   Prepare the cabbage.
5   Prepare the lemon sauce.
6   Prepare the cake.
7   Cook the cabbage. Cover.
8   Cook the sauce.
9   Reheat the pumpkin and potatoes.
10   Cook the cake. Serve hot, cut into wedges with natural low fat yoghurt.
11   Serve first course while the cake is cooking.

THAT SPECIAL MEAL FOR TWO

Both these quick and easy meals can be prepared with very little notice — an impressive dinner can be on the table within an hour.

Summer:

Avocado with Orange Dressing (p 16)
Plaited Fish (p 64)
Braised Leeks
Cherry Tomatoes
Arranged Fruit Salad (p 132)

Winter:

Grilled Grapefruit (p 22)
Mustard Steaks (p 73)
Mouthwatering Mushrooms (p 111)
Braised Carrots and Celery
Mulled Pears (p 136)

CASUAL DINING FOR FOUR

Deliciously different meal ideas for a relaxed evening with friends or family.

Summer:

Celery Dip with Crackers or Pita Chips (p 22)
Chicken Strudel (p 103)
Spinach Salad with Lemon Dressing (p 122)
Wholemeal Rolls
Strawberry Kebabs

Prepare the kebabs by threading whole strawberries onto kebab sticks. Serve with natural low fat yoghurt if wished.

Winter:

Gingered Carrot Soup (p 29)
Mussels and Pasta (p 66)
French Bread
Scrumble Slice with Coffee (p 147)

Photograph: Cheese Log (p.23), Sesame Chicken (p.102), Tomato and Basil Vinaigre (p.120).

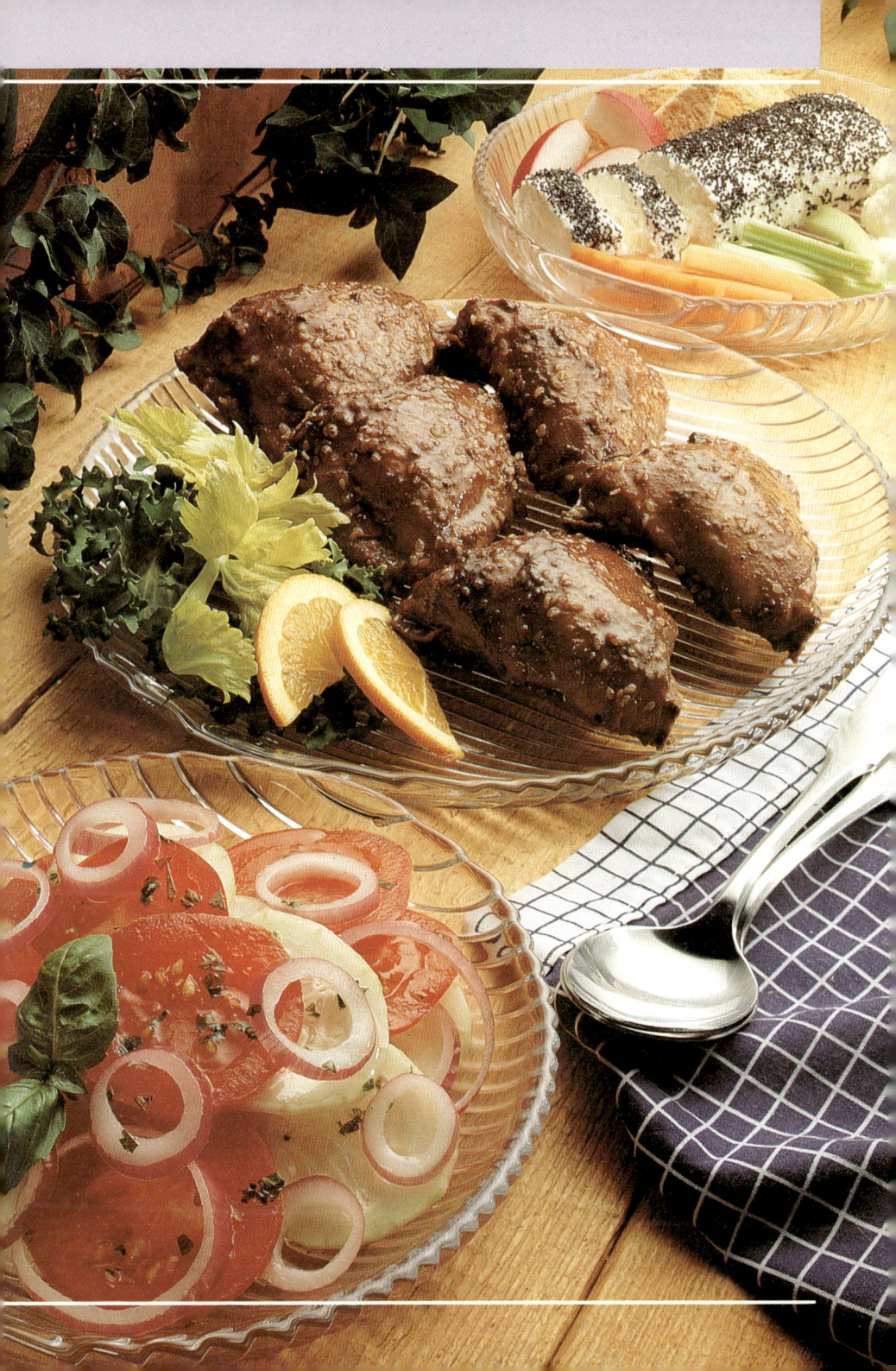

DINNER PARTY FOR SIX

*Simple and attractive ideas for elegant dinner
parties — sure to delight your guests.*

Summer:

Cucumber and Tomato Twin Soup (p 36)
Pineapple and Celery Chicken (p 94)
Pasta Salad with Sesame Dressing (p 118)
Fruit Sorbet (p 138)

Make the sorbet the day before and garnish with
fresh fruit, using the same fruit as is in the sorbet.

Winter:

Chinese Style Soup (p 27)
Fish Fillets with Gooseberry Sauce (p 58)
Sunflower Seed Beans (p 112)
Duchess Potatoes
Caramelised Oranges (p 138)

For Duchess Potatoes, pipe mashed potato into
swirls onto a baking tray. Bake at 200° C for 10-15
minutes or until golden brown.

EASY OUTDOOR EATING (for 6-8 people)

The combination of food we have chosen makes a wonderful picnic — a great way to entertain family or friends either at home or at the beach.

Menu One
Bacon and Garlic Dip with Pita Chips (p 17)
Chicken and Celery Loaf (p 92)
Carrot and Poppyseed Salad (p 121)
Curried Potato Salad (p 119)
Lettuce Salad
Cuppa Square (p 150)
Fresh Fruit

Menu Two
Tandoori Chicken (p 90)
50:50 Rice Salad (p 125)
Lettuce Salad
Wholemeal Rolls
Oaty Fruit Biscuits (p 156)
Fresh Fruit

Menu Three — Barbeque
Cheese Log with crudites (p 23)
Beef Kebabs (p 72)
Sesame Chicken (p 102)
Bean Salad (p 126)
Lettuce Salad
Tomato and Basil Vinaigre (p 120)
French Bread
Banana Coffee Pie (p 139)

BRUNCH

*A relaxing and popular way to entertain friends.
What better welcome than the smell of freshly
baked bread and muffins.*

Freshly squeezed orange or grapefruit juice
Quick Kibbled Wheat Bread (p 153) with
a selection of homemade jams
Blueberry Muffins (p 152)
Fruit Kebabs served with yoghurt
and chopped nuts (p 170)

And if your guests linger longer . . .

Broccoli Stacks (p 40)
Garden Green Salad (p 128)

Photograph: Italian Pasta (p.44).

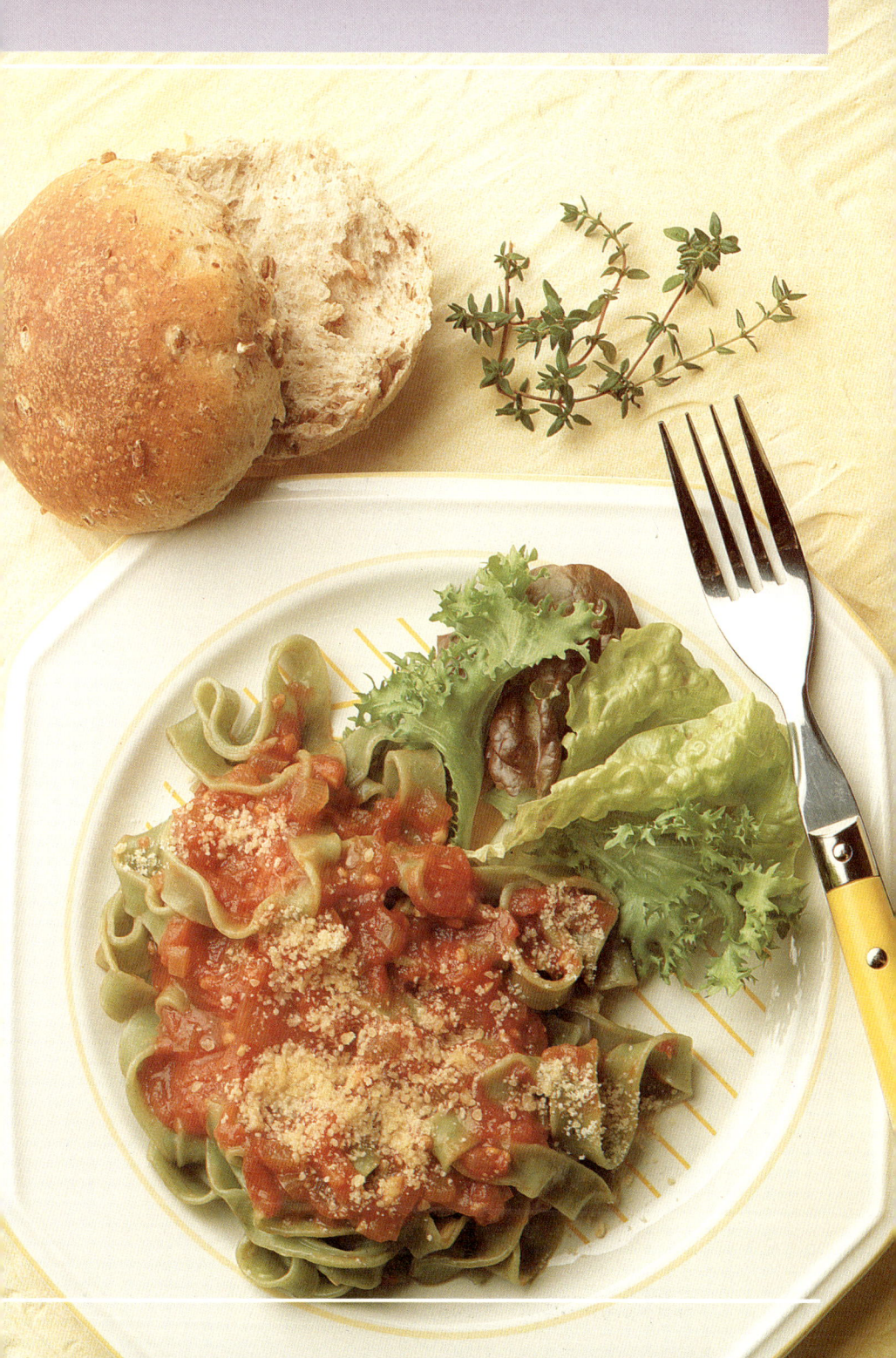

INDEX

D

E

F

L

M

N

INDEX

O

P

Q

R

S

INDEX